The
Pain
Manual

PRINCIPLES
AND
ISSUES
IN
CANCER
PAIN
MANAGEMENT

PEGASUS HEALTHCARE
INTERNATIONAL

The publisher wishes to express its gratitude to Purdue Pharma for an education grant which has made the publication of this book possible.

1st Printing, June 1997
2nd Printing, April 1998
3rd Printing, April 1999
4th Printing, November 2000

Canadian Cataloguing in Publication Data

Librach, S. Lawrence
The pain manual: principles and issues in cancer pain management.
Issued also in French under title: Le manuel de la douleur.
Includes bibliographical references and index.
ISBN 1-895995-13-2
1. Cancer pain—Treatment. 2. Cancer Pain—Chemotherapy.
3. Cancer—Complications—Treatment.
I. Squires, Bruce P. II. Canadian Cancer Society III. Canadian Association of Nurses in Oncology. IV. Title.

RB127.L52 1996   616.99'4061   C96-900632-2

Published by: Pegasus Healthcare International
            A division of Pegasus Communications Inc.

1456 Sherbrooke Street West	King West Centre
3rd Floor	2 Pardee, Suite 203
Montréal, Québec	Toronto, Ontario
H3G lK4	M6K 3H5

The
Pain
Manual

Table of Contents

Foreword

Pain is no stranger to anyone, but just because we have experienced pain does not mean that we are able to understand what it is like when pain is constant. It is especially difficult for health-care professionals who, too often, have been taught to fear that long-term administration of narcotic drugs leads inevitably to undesirable addiction. The consequences have been devastating. Patients have been forced to endure long periods of pain severe enough to jeopardize their comfort, work, sleep and relationships. Many patients with cancer still spend their last days in unnecessary agony, while their families stand helplessly by.

In this revised edition of his popular manual, Dr. Larry Librach provides the most up-to-date outline of the basic and important strategies for managing chronic and increasing pain. He also has added chapters on the management of pain in children and in those with conditions other than cancer. While providing specific regimens and alternatives for using analgesic medications, he also reminds us throughout that analgesics alone are not enough. Appropriate management must encompass the entire patient, how he or she experiences and responds to pain, the psychologic and social effects on both patient and family and how the patient perceives quality of life. How pain is managed must not be the decision of the attending physician alone; the patient, family, all caregivers, and consulting specialists must constitute an open and honest team that responds to the patient's needs and wishes, and the changing nature of the pain.

In revising this edition, Dr. Librach had the expert advice of a superb medical advisory board, the endorsement of the Canadian Cancer Society, the Canadian Association of Nurses in Oncology, and an educational grant from Purdue Frederick.

Bruce P. Squires, MD, PhD
General Editor

Introduction

> *"For all the happiness mankind can gain*
> *Is not in pleasure, but in rest from pain."*
>
> John Dryden, 1631-1700

Five years following the publication of the first edition of *The Pain Manual*, the problem of poorly-controlled pain in cancer patients still occurs all too frequently. Also, new therapies and new formulations of drugs have appeared and improvements on previous treatment regimens have been developed. All have been included in this revised edition. Important chapters on pain in children and treatment of chronic non-malignant pain, as well as information on pain in patients with AIDS/HIV disease have been added.

The treatment of patients in pain still has no magic bullet. To be successful, it depends on careful and diligent attention paid to patient and family concerns and suffering, the basic principles of pain management and the prudent use of analgesics, adjuvant medications and other treatment modalities.

1 Cancer and Pain

According to a review of a number of studies, at least 70 percent of patients with advanced cancer have pain, although the prevalence seems to vary depending on the patients studied.[1]

Pain of some sort is sometimes the first sign of cancer, but in the early stages of the disease it is less common and rarely overwhelming. Pain is very common and often severe in patients with progressive or advanced cancer. Indeed, some hospice programs have reported that 90 percent of their patients have pain. Even seemingly well-functioning ambulatory cancer patients may have significant amounts of severe pain.[2] The critical point is that this frequent and sometimes severe symptom requires prompt and suitable treatment.

Although the figures on prevalence of pain in cancer are important, the worldwide concern that cancer pain has been poorly managed is much more important. The World Health Organization estimates that 80 percent of the five million who die from cancer annually die with uncontrolled pain.[3]

Why is Pain Managed So Poorly?

Several factors account for the often poor management of cancer patients' pain by health professionals:

- lack of knowledge about pain, especially its assessment and treatment;
- biases and fears about the use of opioid (narcotic) analgesics;
- failure to give priority to symptoms in the disease-centered model of care;
- lack of exposure to appropriate clinical role models;
- failure to consider the model of "total pain";
- lack of consultation and treatment resources for pain control.

Also, patient and family factors contribute to the poor management of cancer pain:

■ fear of side effects, especially constipation, sedation and confusion;

■ concerns about addiction;

■ lack of awareness that cancer pain can be treated effectively;

■ a wide variety of communication problems, especially a failure to communicate pain effectively to service providers;

■ concern that the use of strong opioids early on will leave nothing to try if pain worsens;

■ concerns that opioids represent "the end".

These factors are at long last being addressed because of increasing concern about pain among cancer specialists, other physicians and health professionals, patients and families and because of the increasing influence of the palliative-care approach to managing cancer pain.

The Role of Palliative Care

Palliative or hospice care emerged in Britain over 25 years ago, and has been evolving ever since. This new discipline is based on a well-justified concern that the needs of dying patients and their families are not being met by the established health-care system. The hospice movement is now widespread in the developed world.

Although palliative care is not the primary focus of this handbook, its philosophy is essential to the management of pain in cancer patients. The Canadian Palliative Care Association recently defined palliative care:

Palliative care, as a philosophy of care, is the combination of active and compassionate therapies intended to comfort and support individuals and families who are living with a life-threatening illness. During periods of illness and bereavement, palliative care strives to meet physical, psychological, social and spiritual expectations and needs, while remaining sensitive to personal, cul-

tural and religious values, beliefs and practices. Palliative care may be combined with therapies aimed at reducing or curing the illness, or it may be the total focus of care.

Palliative care is planned and delivered through the collaborative efforts of an interdisciplinary team including the individual, family, caregivers and service providers. It should be available to the individual and his/her family at any time during the illness trajectory and bereavement.

While many service providers may be able to deliver some of the therapies that provide comfort and support, the services of a specialized palliative care program may be required as the degree of distress, discomfort and dysfunction increases.

Integral to effective palliative care is the provision of opportunity and support for the caregivers and service providers to work through their own emotions and grief related to the care they are providing.[4]

Palliative care is committed to improving the quality of care for all dying patients through:

- addressing the physical, psychosocial and spiritual needs of dying patients and their families;
- providing person-centered care;
- focusing on the family as the unit of care;
- involving patients and their families at all levels of medical decision-making;
- providing home care;
- using multidisciplinary teams to provide care;
- maintaining excellent communications;
- fostering education and research in the area of caring for dying patients.

These basic commitments will be reflected throughout this manual on pain control in patients with cancer or other terminal illnesses. The holistic approach, which embodies the whole person and the diverse personal, social and environmental factors that affect him or her, should be the "gold standard" for all medical treatment of cancer patients.

Total Pain

Experts, including Saunders[5] and Twycross and Lack,[6] have used the concept of "total pain" to explain that patients' experience of pain is related not only to somatic factors but also to the many other factors that affect their psychologic state. Therefore, to be effective, the treatment of pain must encompass all the factors. The following model of "total pain" represents a further development of the original concept.

The components of "total pain" include the following:

1. **Somatic source.** The pain is produced by a somatic source or sources. Appropriate treatment of pain must be directed at the specific source of the pain as well as at the pain itself. Pain is also influenced by the other common physical symptoms affecting patients with cancer. Physical pain must be addressed before focusing on the assessment of psychologic and family factors and support.

2. **Patients' emotional status.** Patients' emotional status may have considerable effect on the pain that they feel and how they express it. Anger, anxiety, depression and guilt all have a significant effect on pain and must be addressed. The meaning of pain for patients learned through previous experience also strongly affects their emotional response to pain.

3. **Patients' personality.** Patients' basic personality may influence how they experience the pain. Poor self-esteem, inability to discuss and express emotions, significant personality disorders, etc., may have a deleterious effect on patients' experience of pain and how they respond to treatment.

4. **Patients' family.** There is now considerable evidence that the family and its relationship to the patient have major effects on many different types of illness. This is especially obvious in managing patients with pain. Compliance, health beliefs, family dynamics, family dysfunction and other issues will influence patients' expression of pain and their response to treatment.

5. **Patient and family ecology.** This phrase refers to basic issues of education, economic status and resources, social supports, history of illnesses and religion. A major factor in both the expression of pain and response to treatment may lie in the patient's and family's cultural or ethnic origins. Service providers working in unfamiliar cultural settings must try to understand the family's health beliefs. Difficulties may arise when unwitting prejudices, biases and stereotypes interfere with treatment.

6. **Service providers.** Patients' experience and expression of pain and their response to treatment are strongly influenced by the environment created by the health-care team. Team members' biases and fears may have considerable impact on the pain. Previous negative experiences with service providers and institutions will definitely have an undesirable influence on patients' pain.

Total pain can be compared to an ameba whose shape changes constantly, as illustrated in Figure 1. At various times, it will appear differently and the component factors may vary in effect on the pain and its expression. The most effective approach to a patient's pain will include consideration of ALL the factors underlying "total pain". An approach that considers only the somatic source will expose the patient to needless suffering. Conversely, an approach based entirely on psychosocial support does nothing to help patients with severe physical pain.

Figure 1: Total Pain

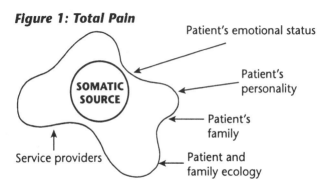

References

1. Bonica JJ. Treatment of cancer pain: current status and future needs. In: Fields HL, Dubner R, Cervero F (eds.), *Advances in Pain Research and Therapy*, Vol. 9, Raven Press, New York 1985.

2. Portenoy RK, Miransky, J. Thaler et al. Pain in ambulatory patients with lung and colon cancer. *Cancer* 1992; 70:1616-24.

3. World Health Organization Technical Report No. 804. *Cancer Pain and Palliative Care*. Geneva, 1990.

4. Ferris FD, Cummings I (eds.). *Palliative Care: Towards a Consensus in Standardized Principles of Practice*. Canadian Palliative Care Association, Ottawa 1995; 12.

5. Saunders CM (ed). *The Management of Terminal Disease*. Edward Arnold, London 1978; 194-5.

6. Twycross RW, Lack S. *Symptom Control in Far Advanced Cancer: Pain Relief*. Pitman, London 1984.

2 Cancer Pain: Causes and Classification

The causes and classification of pain are important to the clinical management of cancer pain.

The Basic Physiology of Pain

Physicians and other service providers sometimes have a very simplistic model of pain, in which the pain experience is reduced to a noxious peripheral stimulus to a nerve ending, causing messages to be carried directly to the brain to produce cerebral awareness of pain. Pain is, in fact, a very complex physiologic event. The exact components of the neural pathway and the neurologic events that produce the experience of pain are neither totally known nor within the scope of this manual. But several features are important to understanding treatment options.

- Different types of nerve fibres carry peripheral pain messages. These nerve fibres are stimulated by tissue injury and by the release of chemical mediators.

- Pain impulses are modulated at all levels by efferent and afferent impulses. A major site for this modulation occurs in the dorsal horn of the spinal cord.

- Pain fibres generally cross to the opposite side and are usually carried to higher levels via the lateral spinothalamic tracts of the spinal cord, thence to the thalamus and cortical centers. However, other pathways for pain transmission exist, although the exact interactions and functions of these pathways are not completely known.

- Special inhibitory neurotransmitters such as ß-endorphins, enkephalin and dynorphin bind to the same opiate receptors as exogenous opioids and exert similar effects. These compounds block the ability of neurotransmitters to activate pain pathways.

- The influence of higher central nervous system centres in the brain is not completely known; however, we do know that fears, attitudes and emotions all affect pain experience and that chronic pain will produce anxiety and depression.

- Pain threshold, the least experience of pain that a person can recognize, varies widely from person to person and generally is not a clinically measurable or useful concept. Pain tolerance is the greatest level of pain a person is prepared to tolerate. Both pain threshold and pain tolerance will be influenced by many factors: physiologic factors, previous pain experiences, family factors and attitudes of service providers and caregivers. Irrespective of the patient's pain threshold or tolerance, the pain must be treated.

The complexity of pain experiences accounts for the variability in the expression of pain and of the responses to different treatments.

Causes of Cancer Pain

Pain in cancer patients often originates from several causes, and it is important to discriminate among them. Pain from different causes may require somewhat different therapeutic approaches. Most pain in cancer is a result of the destructive and invasive effects of cancer but other causes need to be considered. Table 1 summarizes the common causes of pain in cancer.

Only one-quarter of patients will have just one type of pain. Up to one-third of patients will have four or more different types of pain.

Table 1: Common Causes of Pain in Cancer Patients

Caused by the Cancer	Bone infiltration with or without muscle spasm
	Nerve compression, infiltration or destruction
	Visceral involvement
	Soft tissue infiltration
	Ulceration with or without infection
	Raised intracranial pressure
Related to Therapy	Constipation
	Postoperative acute pain
	Postoperative chronic neuropathic pain
	Phantom limb pain
	Postradiation inflammation, fibrosis or neuritis
	Postradiation myelopathy
	Chemotherapy-induced peripheral neuropathy
	Bone necrosis from radiotherapy
Related to the Cancer	Muscle spasm
	Constipation
	Bedsores
	Lymphedema
	Candidiasis
	Herpetic neuralgia
	Deep vein thrombosis
	Pulmonary embolus
	Limb ischemia
Unrelated to Either the Cancer or its Treatment	Musculoskeletal pain
	Headache
	Constipation
	Arthritis
	Ischemic cardiac pain

Pain Classification

Clinical classification of cancer pain has important management ramifications. Basically, pain can be separated into nociceptive pain, neuropathic pain, mixed pain and pain of unknown origin. Nociceptive pain is caused by tissue damage created by pressure, infiltration or destruction by an identifiable somatic or visceral lesion. Neuropathic pain is caused by pressure, invasion or destruction of peripheral or central nervous tissues, which leads to complex and abnormal spinal cord or thalamic neural processes that produce sustained pain. The diagnosis of neuropathic pain relies on special features in the pain history, evidence of nerve damage and clinical suspicion because of the anatomic location of the cancer. Pain in many instances is a combination of nociceptive and neuropathic pain. Infrequently, the cause of pain may not be exactly identified despite appropriate investigations.

The classification, examples and potential specific management issues are detailed in Table 2, p. 18.

Pain has been classified according to how it responds to opioids but the classification was oversimplified. For example, nociceptive pain was usually classified as opioid-responsive while neuropathic pain was often described as opioid-resistant. It is now known that this is not the case.[1] Physiologic mechanisms such as changes in opiate receptors, abnormal and unregulated firing of axons and changes in neurotransmitters may be responsible for relatively lower levels of opioid responsiveness. However, there is no absolute way of predicting whether a patient's pain will be responsive or resistant to opioids. Responsiveness to opioids also depends on the various factors outlined under "total pain" in Chapter 1 (p. 11). Physiologic factors such as absorption and drug metabolism also may affect a particular patient's response. Therefore, a clinical trial of opioids is warranted in all these pain syndromes.

The search for the cause or causes of pain may reveal the pathway to specific treatment, but it cannot be used as an absolute guide to therapy.

Table 2: Clinical Classification of Pain

TYPE	CLINICAL EXAMPLE	SPECIFIC TREATMENT POSSIBILITIES
Nociceptive Pain		
Superficial somatic	Skin invasion or ulceration	Opioid analgesics Glucocorticosteroids Drugs for neuropathic pain Antibiotics
Deep somatic—bone	Bone metastases Pathologic fractures	Opioid analgesics, NSAIDs Radiotherapy, surgery, chemotherapy
Deep somatic—muscle, soft tissue	Muscle invasion Soft tissue masses	Opioid analgesics Radiotherapy, chemotherapy
Visceral	Hepatomegaly Bladder spasms	Opioid analgesics, glucocorticosteroids Radiotherapy, chemotherapy Antispasmodics Neurolytic procedures
Raised intracranial pressure	Brain tumors Meningeal carcinomatosis	Glucocorticosteroids, radiotherapy Opioid analgesics
Neuropathic Pain		
	Pelvic tumor invading lumbosacral plexus Brachial plexus invasion Spinal cord compression	Opioid analgesics Antidepressants Anticonvulsants Glucocorticosteroids
Mixed	Pancreatic pain from posterior invasion of a vertebra and local spinal nerve roots	Combination therapy aimed at both neuropathic and nociceptive pain
Unknown	Persistent pain, the cause of which cannot be determined by history and investigations	Opioid analgesics or adjuncts, or both

Reference

1.   Portenoy R. Drug therapy for cancer pain. *J Hospice Palliative Care* 1992; (Nov/Dec):22-31.

3 *Pain Assessment*

Basic Guidelines

Assessment of the patient's pain is the critical first step to effective pain management; it requires careful attention to four basic guidelines.

- **Listen carefully and trust the patient's assessment of pain.** *Pain* can be defined as whatever the patient says hurts. The best judge of a patient's pain is the patient.[1] The need to rely almost entirely on the patient's report of pain without more "objective" evidence accounts for some of the reluctance of service providers and, perhaps, even of the patient's family to believe the patient's account.

- **Observe and recognize the typical pictures of chronic distress.** *Chronic pain* differs remarkably from acute pain because it does not have some of the obvious physiologic sequelae and body language that characterizes acute pain. Patients rarely show the typical picture of distress associated with, for example, fractured bones or acute abdominal emergencies (Figure 2, p. 20).

  Caregivers who think they can estimate the severity of a patient's pain by simple visual inspection not only delude themselves, but also constitute a major reason why pain is treated poorly. For example, patients with chronic pain can often sleep most of the night even though their sleep may be disturbed and uncomfortable. But nurses or family members may not wake a patient for middle-of-the-night doses of analgesic because they believe that sleep means the patient has no pain.

- **Employ the concept of total pain.** *Total pain* and the diverse factors that influence it may mislead caregivers into trying to determine how much pain is "physical" and how much is "psychologic". There is truly no way to differentiate pain on this basis; the division between "organic" and "psychologic" pain is as artificial as the separation of mind and body. Pain is always subjective and individual.

Figure 2: Typical Pictures of Acute and Chronic Pain

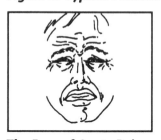

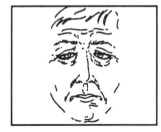

The Face of Acute Pain

Physicians are usually trained to recognize and treat the acute pain of emergency rooms. Here the face reveals hyperactivity of the autonomic nervous system (sweating, pallor, tachycardia, hypertension). The face of acute pain is grimacing, crying, anxious.

The Face of Chronic Pain

In sharp contrast, the face of the patient with chronic pain shows very few signs of distress. Autonomic signs are absent. Often the suffering is hidden beneath a brave, stoic face. After long periods of unrelieved pain, the face no longer reveals anxiety but exhaustion and depression. The lack of objective signs and the depressed, sleepy face is often misinterpreted and the patient's complaints of severe pain discounted. Facial grimacing cannot be used as an indicator of pain intensity. Learn to recognize and treat the face of both acute and chronic pain.

Reproduced from *Cancer Pain: A Monograph on the Management of Cancer.* Health and Welfare Canada, Minister of Supply and Services 1984, p. 11. With permission.

■   Use external measurement tools individually. *Pain intensity and quality are difficult to measure exactly.* Pain questionnaires and scales are useful in following patients. But there are no physiologic measurements to assess pain. In a health-care system that values accurate diagnosis and assessment, this lack of objective measurement undermines physicians' and nurses' confidence in basing treatment on what patients say about their pain, and may lead to poor treatment. Again, pain is always subjective and individual.

The Pain History

A thorough review of the history of the pain is the first assessment step. It is the responsibility of not only the physician, but also nurses and other members of the health-care team. If taken accurately and without bias, the pain history will give valuable clues to the causes of the pain or pains and point the way to appropriate treatment.

- The pain history should be taken in a relaxed setting and with careful attention paid to the patient's comfort and position.

- In most cases, the person taking the history should sit comfortably beside the patient at the same eye level. The body language conveyed by standing over a patient at the bedside (a position of authority or dominance) may interfere with obtaining some aspects of the history, especially the more sensitive psychosocial aspects.

- Questions should be open-ended and the patient should be encouraged to supply as many descriptive words about the pain as are possible. Very frail patients may require some prompting with more leading questions, but leading questions should be avoided, if possible, with most others. If, during the interview, the patient exhibits a dominant emotion, especially anger or severe anxiety, it must be acknowledged and at least partially dealt with before any further probing is done.

- It is often helpful to have a family member present during the history-taking to corroborate the patient's history of pain. This may also reveal the family's acceptance (or non-acceptance) of the pain problem and familial issues that may factor into the appropriate management of the pain.

Describing Pain

Questions to ask should include those about onset, location, duration, severity, radiation, and relieving and aggravating factors. Because cancer patients often have more than one type of pain, the patients' description of each pain should be carefully assessed.

- **Somatic pain: Bone and muscle pain** is:
  - relatively well localized;
  - worse on movement;
  - tender to pressure over the area;
  - often accompanied by a dull background aching pain;
  - sometimes referred, if it is bone pain, but not along dermatomes; e.g., hip pain to the knee.

- **Superficial somatic pain from skin invasion or multiple subcutaneous nodules** is often:
  - well localized to the superficial skin area;
  - itching or burning in quality.

- **Visceral pain** is:
  - often poorly localized, deep and aching;
  - usually constant;
  - often referred; e.g., diaphragmatic irritation may be referred to the right shoulder, pelvic visceral pain is often referred to the sacral or perineal area.

- **Neuropathic pain** may be manifested by:
  - a burning, deeply aching quality that may be accompanied by some sudden, sharp lancinating pain;
  - often a dermatomal or peripheral nerve distribution or radiation;
  - numbness or tingling over the area;
  - hyperesthesia over an area of skin;
  - severe pain from even slight pressure from clothing or light touch (allodynia);
  - usually constant and severe pain often preceding the development of objective neurologic findings.

- **Severity of pain** is important and patients should be asked to rate it, perhaps using one of the scales described in this chapter (p. 24).

- **How pain affects daily living** is an important part of the history. The time a patient spends at rest because of the pain is a good indicator of its severity. Pain will often affect appetite, although anorexia is also a common symptom of cancer. Activities at work or at home will be decreased and, although they may sleep, patients in pain often report the sleep to be fitful, disturbed and unrestorative.

- **Past medications.** The person taking the history should also delve into the patient's response to past treatment. Questions have to be asked about current and past medications—how much, how often, the maximum effect, the duration of effect and related side effects. The use of other pain treatments such as massage, acupuncture, transcutaneous electrical nerve stimulation (TENS), heat, cold and alternative therapies needs to be assessed.

- **Fears about the pain and about opioid analgesics** must be explored. Cultural attitudes toward pain and its treatment are also important. A psychosocial history is important at this stage. Some understanding of the family and of its resources and dynamics should be acquired over several interviews and will, of course, make the care plan more appropriate and acceptable to both patient and family.

- **A survey of other symptoms** is important; symptoms such as constipation and nausea may be overlooked and yet they can play a major role in the production of pain and response to treatment.

It is easy to obtain most information about the pain at a single interview, but information from other caregivers, if available, needs to be gathered to make the assessment as complete as possible. Information should be carefully recorded in the patient's interdisciplinary health record. A body chart will often help in documenting the locations of different pains.

Pain Assessment Tools

There are several ways of trying to quantify the intensity of a patient's pain. Pain questionnaires such as the McGill Pain Questionnaire[2] are important research tools, but they are often impractical and difficult to administer in the clinical situation where several caregivers are involved and patients are often too ill to handle a lengthy inquiry.

The most practical assessment tool is the visual or verbal analog scale. Several are in common use. All have descriptors such as "little or no pain" at one end and "excruciating pain" or "the most severe pain imaginable" at the other. Patients find it extremely easy to quantify their pain on a 5- or 10-point scale (Figure 3).

One such approach, the Edmonton Symptom Assessment Scales (ESAS),[3,4] uses visual or verbal analog scales and other pictorial or graphic representations to monitor the progress of pain and other symptoms (Appendix A, p. 106).

Figure 3: Example of a Visual Analog Scale for Pain

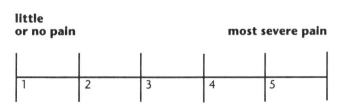

These scales are simple for service providers to administer and are easily understood by families. The results are interpretable for one patient but cannot be used to compare a patient's with other patients' pain.

A pain diary is helpful, especially for patients at home. A sample of a simple pain report form is included in Appendix A (p. 106).

These pain assessment tools—diary and analog scale— are also useful in evaluating the effectiveness of pharmacologic or other therapy.

It is hoped that new staging systems for pain such as the Edmonton Staging System for Cancer Pain[4] will provide a more rigorous structure to the assessment and description of pain.

Investigating Wisely

The last point to be emphasized is the appropriate use of investigations in assessing pain in patients with advanced cancer. No investigation is 100 percent sensitive or 100 percent specific. For instance, bone scans to identify bone metastases are often but not always correct. Radiological investigations are not definitive enough in most cases to confirm all sources of pain. Laboratory investigation is often not helpful.

Pain in cancer patients should be treated before the results of investigations are known. Leaving patients needlessly in pain for days or weeks while awaiting the results of tests is inhumane. There is little risk to early treatment, and medication can always be decreased or stopped if another more definitive treatment such as radiotherapy is successful.

Patients with advanced disease should be spared unnecessary repeated investigations. Increase in tumor size and increase in size and numbers of metastases may provide little useful information in managing the patient's symptoms and suffering, and such information is often demoralizing to patients and families. Repeated investigations will also use up considerable patient energy and may cause pain themselves.

References

1.   McCaffery M, Beebe A. *A Clinical Manual for Nursing Practice*. CV Mosby, Toronto 1989, p. 6-33.

2.   Melzack, R. *McGill Pain Questionnaire: Major Properties and Scoring Methods*. Elsevier, Amsterdam 1975.

3.   Bruera E, Kuehn N, Miller MJ et al. The Edmonton Symptom Assessment Scale: A simple method for the assessment of palliative care patients. *J Palliative Care* 1991; 7(2):6-9.

4.   Bruera E, Schoeller T, Wenk R et al. A prospective multicentre assessment of the Edmonton Staging system for cancer pain. *J Pain Sympt Manage* 1995; 10:348-55.

4 Basic Principles of Effective Pain Control

Attention to four sets of basic principles assures the most effective control of the patient's pain.

General Principles

- **Always remembering the concept of "total pain".** It is the key to successful control of pain.

- **Having a commitment to pain management.** This is an essential commitment by individual health professionals, institutions and community agencies.

- **Educating the patient, family and other service providers and involving them in the pain treatment plan.** The effective care team includes a trusting patient and family. Considerable patient and family learning is required to understand pain assessment and describe realistic pain-control objectives, the treatment and potential adverse effects. Service providers also need to deal with fears about opioids, explore other needs, describe the monitoring of the pain, and outline the responsibilities of all. This process should involve at least one family conference. Supportive literature about cancer pain is available (Appendix B, p. 109). A written care plan, for all to see, is invaluable. Lines of communication should be clearly established so that patient and family can obtain help quickly.

- **Using an interdisciplinary approach.** Clinical experience in pain management has shown that an interdisciplinary team approach is more effective than others in dealing with the wide variety of issues that constitute "total pain" and in using adjuvant therapies to maximum advantage.

- **Being flexible.** There are no uniformly successful formulas for pain control. The physician and other caregivers must avoid rigid treatment regimens that, for instance, have upper limits of opioid dosages or have no room for complementary treatments, such as relaxation therapy and therapeutic touch. Treatment must always be individualized.

- **Asking for help.** One must not be afraid to ask for help. Palliative- or hospice-care resources are increasingly available. Help can be just a telephone call away if the patient's pain and other symptoms are not controlled (Appendix B, p. 109).

Principles of Assessment

- **Doing a thorough but relatively rapid assessment of the pain.** The most important skill the physician and other team members can bring to a pain assessment is listening carefully to the patient's story of the pain and other relevant aspects—physical, psychologic, social and spiritual—of the total pain experience.

- **Investigating wisely.** Investigations should be limited to those that could make a difference to management of the pain. If the diagnostic test will not alter the treatment already planned, why do the test?

- **Avoiding unnecessary delay in treating the pain, especially if it is severe.** Delay causes unjustifiable suffering. Just as antibiotics should not be withheld from a patient with severe infection while the physician waits for the results of cultures, analgesics, including strong opioids, should not be withheld from a patient in pain.

Principles of Analgesic Therapy

- **Following a stepped approach to analgesia that depends on the severity of the pain.** The World Health Organization,[1] The Canadian Expert Advisory Committee,[2] the American Pain Society,[3] the U.S. Department of Health and Human Services[4] and other authorities have recommended a stepped approach to pain relief (Figure 4).

The stepped approach has scientific validity,[5] but patients in severe pain can be treated from the beginning with strong opioids and the first steps are not necessary.

■ **Giving medication orally whenever possible.** In most cases, analgesics can be given orally. Alternative routes of analgesic administration may be required in certain circumstances (see Chapter 10, p. 73).

■ **Constant pain requires regular administration of analgesics to maintain constant levels of analgesia.** The preferred regimen comprises regular doses of oral analgesics. Regular dosing, according to the duration of the analgesic effect, avoids the peaks of pain and, often, the peaks of side effects associated with p.r.n. prescriptions.

■ **Consideration should be given to adjuvant therapy at all stages.** This may include surgery, radiation, chemotherapy, adjuvant drugs and other supportive methods.

Figure 4: World Health Organization Analgesic Stepped Approach in Cancer Pain Relief

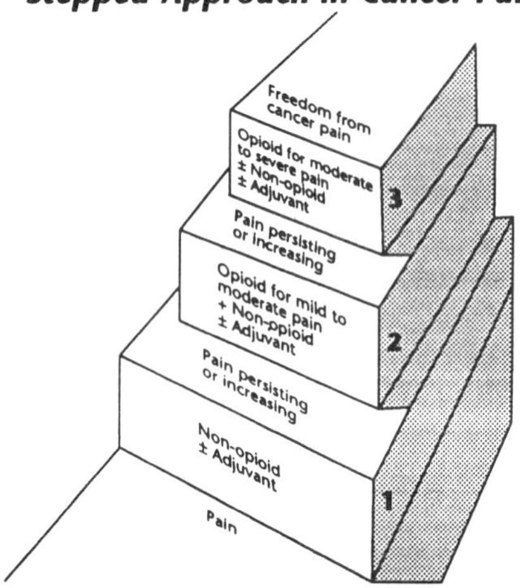

Freedom from cancer pain

Opioid for moderate to severe pain ± Non-opioid ± Adjuvant **3**

Pain persisting or increasing

Opioid for mild to moderate pain + Non-opioid ± Adjuvant **2**

Pain persisting or increasing

Non-opioid ± Adjuvant **1**

Pain

Adapted from *WHO Draft Interim Guidelines Handbook on Relief of Cancer Pain*, World Health Organization, Geneva, 1990.

- **Always leaving instructions for a "breakthrough" dose** (p. 50). Breakthrough pain occurs relatively frequently in most cancer patients with pain. It is defined as an increase above the baseline level in pain that may require a supplemental or "rescue" dose of opioid to return stability to pain control. Breakthrough pain may signal just a variation in the pain or it may signal a worsening of pain or new factors contributing to pain.

- **Anticipating and preventing adverse effects of analgesics.** Successful pain management requires an aggressive and preventive approach to side effects of analgesics and other treatments.

- **Treating other symptoms, such as constipation, nausea and muscle spasm aggressively.** These may exacerbate the patient's pain (see Chapter 9, p. 63).

Principles of Monitoring

- **Monitoring the patient frequently, and keeping in touch.** Patients require frequent monitoring of their pain and their response to treatment, especially at the beginning of pain-control efforts. Patients and family should understand the pain assessment tools and be involved in making appropriate written records. If the patient is at home, daily phone calls may be required. If the pain is severe, analgesic orders should be assessed at least every 12 to 18 hours. Patients should not be sent home with newly prescribed medication without early and timely follow-up.

- **Communicating effectively with other service providers.** An effective pain management plan includes effective communication with all members of the interdisciplinary team. Home-care nurses have an important role in monitoring patients at home.

References

1. World Health Organization. *Cancer Pain Relief.* World Health Organization Office of Publications, Geneva 1990.

2. *Cancer Pain: A Monograph on the Management of Cancer Pain. A report of the Expert Advisory Committee on the Management of Severe Chronic Pain in Cancer Patients.* Health and Welfare Canada, Minister of Supply and Services 1984, p. 20.

3. *Principles of Analgesic Use in the Treatment of Acute Pain and Cancer Pain.* 3rd ed. American Pain Society, 1992.

4. *Management of Cancer Pain. Clinical Practice Guidelines.* U.S. Department of Health and Human Services. Public Health Service, Agency for Health Care Policy and Research, 1994.

5. Ventafridda V, Tamburini M, Caraceni A et al. A validation study of the WHO method for cancer pain relief. *Cancer* 1987; 59:850-6.

5 Non-Opioid Analgesic Drugs

Non-opioid analgesics are generally used in the treatment of cancer patients with mild to moderate pain and have specific applications in the treatment of bone pain (p. 35). The non-opioid drugs include acetylsalicylic acid (ASA) and non-acetylated salicylates, other non-steroidal anti-inflammatory drugs (NSAIDs) and acetaminophen.

ASA and Non-Acetylated Salicylates

The salicylates are important members of the class of non-opioid drugs. ASA is the most widely used.

- **Mechanism of action.** How salicylates work is not exactly known. Acetylsalicylic acid inhibits prostaglandin synthesis peripherally, thereby exerting anti-inflammatory and analgesic effects. Non-acetylated salicylates are much weaker inhibitors of prostaglandin synthesis. All salicylates may inhibit neutrophils and this may account for the anti-inflammatory activity.[1]

- **Pharmacokinetics.** Salicylates are very well absorbed from the upper gastrointestinal tract. They are metabolized in the liver and excreted in the urine. Half-lives vary according to preparations: ASA has the shortest; diflunisal, the longest.

Table 3: Recommended Dosages of Salicylates

GENERIC NAME	DOSAGE
Acetylsalicylic acid (ASA) *	650 mg q4h to q6h for pain or fever
	975 mg q6h for anti-inflammatory effect
Choline magnesium salicylate†	500 mg t.i.d. to 1.5 gm b.i.d.
Diflunisal	250 to 500 mg q12h

*enteric-coated preparations are recommended
†fewer gastrointestinal effects, lesser effect on platelet function compared with ASA[2]

- **Adverse effects.** The most common are gastrointestinal: epigastric distress, heartburn, nausea and vomiting, and gastrointestinal (especially gastric) bleeding. Mucosal damage and microscopic bleeding are almost universal in patients taking salicylates because of local absorption and irritation, as well as systemic effects. Thus, although distress may be reduced by enteric-coated preparations, it is not eliminated. There is evidence that gastrointestinal adverse effects are considerably less common with non-acetylated salicylates compared with ASA.[3]

  Constipation may also occur with salicylates. Other adverse effects include tinnitus, dizziness, vertigo and decreased hearing (especially in the elderly), and serious but infrequent (5 percent) hypersensitivity reactions. There may be cross-sensitivity with other non-steroidal anti-inflammatory drugs.

  Significant drug interactions occur with anticoagulants; therefore, salicylates should always be avoided in the patient who is anticoagulated. ASA also affects platelet function, increasing the risk of bleeding. Non-acetylated salicylates do not affect platelet function. Salicylates are also to be avoided in patients receiving chemotherapy.

  It should also be remembered that salicylates potentiate the effect of hypoglycemic drugs.

Other Non-Steroidal Anti-Inflammatory Drugs (NSAIDs)

In the last 20 years the number and diversity of NSAIDs have increased remarkably. Like salicylates, they have analgesic, antipyretic and anti-inflammatory activities.[4,5] They also share salicylates' many adverse effects.[4,5]

- **Mechanism of action.** The major known action of this diverse group of drugs is thought to involve inhibition of prostaglandin synthesis at peripheral sites of inflammation. However, the analgesic effect is not related to the degree of prostaglandin inhibition. No central action has been demonstrated.

- **Pharmacokinetics.** NSAIDs are generally well absorbed from the upper gastrointestinal tract, and those forms suitable for rectal administration are relatively well absorbed through the rectal mucosa. NSAIDs are metabolized by the liver and excreted mainly in the urine and partly in the bile.

- **Adverse effects.** The major adverse effects are gastrointestinal: heartburn, epigastric distress, ulceration, nausea and vomiting, and gastrointestinal bleeding. They are arguably less severe than those associated with salicylates. Indomethacin may also be associated with depression, confusion and drowsiness, notably in the elderly, although any of the NSAIDs may have some CNS effects. Salt and water retention may cause or worsen edema. NSAIDs may be associated with decreasing renal function, especially in the elderly.

  The major drug interaction to be concerned about with NSAIDs is in patients receiving anticoagulants—again, because of the risk of hemorrhage.

- **Choice of drug.** There is little comparative evidence showing differences in efficacy between the various NSAIDs. NSAIDs have an analgesic ceiling effect whereby giving greater doses does not produce an increased analgesic effect. For severe pain, it is recommended that ceiling doses of NSAIDs be used. Ketorolac has been promoted as an alternative to low-dose opioids such as morphine but gastrointestinal side effects should limit its use orally to 7 days or parenterally to 2 days at the most. Table 4 (p. 34) lists some of the available preparations.

Table 4: Recommended Dosages of Some Common NSAIDs

Generic Name	Dosage
Propionic Acids	
Ibuprofen	200 to 600 mg t.i.d. to q.i.d.
Flurbiprofen	50 to 100 mg b.i.d. or t.i.d.
Ketoprofen[*]	50 to 100 mg b.i.d. or t.i.d.
Naproxen[‡][*]	250 to 375 mg t.i.d.
Tiaprofenic acid[‡]	300 mg b.i.d.
Indoles	
Indomethacin[‡][*]	25 to 50 mg t.i.d.
Sulindac	50 to 100 mg t.i.d.
Acetic Acids	
Tolmetin	200 to 600 mg t.i.d.
Diclofenac[‡][*]	25 to 50 mg t.i.d.
Ketorolac[†]	10 to 30 mg p.o. q4 to 6 h 10 to 30 mg i.m. q4 to 6 h
Oxicams	
Piroxicam[*]	10 to 20 mg q.d.
Tenoxicam	20 mg q.d.

[*] rectal suppository available
[†] the only NSAID with parenteral formulation; only indicated for short-term management, e.g., ≤ 7 days orally, ≤ 2 days parenterally
[‡] controlled-release preparations available

Acetaminophen

A synthetic derivative of the acetanilid group of drugs, acetaminophen has analgesic and antipyretic activities. It does not have the significant gastrointestinal toxicity of NSAIDs and has minimal side effects.[6,7] It can be used by patients who are ASA-sensitive.

■ **Mechanism of action.** Acetaminophen acts peripherally and, perhaps, has some CNS effect, but its mechanism of action is not entirely known. It has little if any effect on prostaglandin synthesis *in vitro*, although it may inhibit synthesis *in vivo*. It seems to have little if any anti-inflammatory activity. Acetaminophen is metabolized in the liver and the metabolites are excreted in the urine. Mild or moderate liver disease does not seem to affect the metabolism of this drug.

■ **Dosage.** The recommended usual dose in adults is 650 mg q4h with the maximal dose being 1000 mg q4h. Dosage forms include tablets, capsules, liquid, and rectal suppositories. Acetaminophen is used very frequently for mild pain in combination with oxycodone and codeine (pp. 42-43).

■ **Adverse effects.** Acetaminophen is virtually free of side effects at the recommended dosage levels. But it does interact somewhat with warfarin, and must be used with some caution in patients taking that anticoagulant. With long-term high dosage, renal or hepatic damage is a possibility. There is minimal chance that the drug, at recommended doses (maximum 4 to 6 gm per day), will have toxic effects on the liver. Liver damage from acetaminophen has not been documented in palliative care literature.

Salicylates and Other NSAIDs in Bone Pain

It is believed that metastases to bone produce pain partly because of the release of prostaglandins; therefore, NSAIDs, because of their inhibition of prostaglandins, have a major role to play in bone pain. Thus, it seems logical to use NSAIDs in the presence of bone pain from metastatic invasion. Response is variable because factors other than the release of prostaglandins may be responsible for the pain. NSAIDs may also be of use in tumors such as lymphoma and myeloma where there has been no evidence of prostaglandin production, and in very inflammatory tumors, such as massive chest wall recurrence of breast cancer.

Radiotherapy must always be considered in bone pain.

Cytoprotective Agents[4,8]

The tendency of NSAIDs to cause adverse gastrointestinal effects limits their use in many patients. The use of H_2-receptor antagonist drugs, such as cimetidine and ranitidine, and of other drugs affecting gastric acid secretion may be effective in preventing duodenal ulceration and bleeding but not the more common gastritis or gastric ulceration and bleeding. Cytoprotective agents should be considered in patients who have shown good response to NSAIDs but experienced gastritis or gastric ulceration. Sucralfate (1 gm q.i.d.) or misoprostol (200 µg q.i.d.) have been shown to reduce gastrointestinal problems when given concurrently with NSAIDs.[9] Misoprostol has significant gastrointestinal effects itself, namely nausea and diarrhea. Misoprostol also has been associated with decreased absorption of indomethacin, but how it affects other NSAIDs is not clear. Cytoprotective agents, of course, further complicate the often complex medication regimens in cancer patients and add considerable cost. *Therefore, routine use of gastric acid suppressants and cytoprotective agents is probably not indicated at present.*

References

1. Altman RD. Neutrophil activation: An alternative to prostaglandin inhibition as the mechanism of action for NSAIDs. *Semin Arthr Rheum* 1990; 4(Suppl 2):1-6.

2. Portenoy R. Drug therapy for cancer pain. *J Hospice Palliative Care.* 1992 (Nov/Dec):22-31.

3. Kilander A, Dotevall G. Endoscopic evaluation of the comparative effects of acetylsalicylic acid and choline magnesium trisalicylate on human gastric and duodenal mucosa. *Br J Rheum* 1983; 22:36-40.

4. Bjarnason I, Macpherson AJS. Intestinal toxicity of non-steroidal anti-inflammatory drugs. *Pharm Ther* 1994; 62:145-57.

5. Lanza LL, Walker AM, Bortnichak EA et al. Peptic ulcer and gastrointestinal hemmorhage associated with nonsteroidal anti-inflammatory drug use in patients younger than 65 years. *Arch Intern Med* 1995; 155:1371-7.

6. Schueler L, Harper JL. Acetaminophen toxicity: Report of case and review of the literature. *J Oral Maxillofac Surg* 1995; 53:1208-12.

7. Blakely P, McDonald BR. Acute renal failure due to acetaminophen ingestion: A case report and review of the literature. *J Am Soc Nephrol* 1995; 6:48-53.

8. Stalnikowicz R, Rachmilewitz D. NSAID-induced gastroduodenal damage: Is prevention needed? A review and metaanalysis. *J Clin Gastroenterol* 1993; 17(3):238-43.

9. Valentini M, Cannizzaro R, Poletti M. Nonsteroidal anti-inflammatory drugs for cancer pain: Comparison between misoprostol and ranitidine in prevention of upper gastrointestinal damage. *J Clin Oncol* 1995; 13:2637-42.

6 Opioid Analgesic Drugs

The opioid or narcotic analgesics are the major drugs used for relieving pain in patients with cancer. Derivatives of the opium poppy, they have been used as analgesics for centuries. However, at the end of the 19th century, the widespread use of medications such as opium, morphine and heroin for all sorts of reasons other than pain led to widespread addiction and, subsequently, restrictive legislation. Abundant myths and fears about opioids have been a major force in preventing adequate control of pain, whatever the cause. If palliative or hospice care has made a contribution to any area of healthcare, it has been in promoting the appropriate use of opioid analgesics.

Basic Pharmacology of Opioid Analgesics

Knowledge of several important pharmacologic features of the opioid drugs will improve clinicians' understanding of their use.

■ Site of action and receptors. Opioids generally suppress neuronal activity. They act at opiate receptors concentrated within certain areas of the central nervous system (CNS); the important ones include the dorsal horn of the spinal cord, the periaqueductal gray matter, and the thalamus. Opiate receptors affecting respiration and vomiting are in the brainstem; those mediating effects on mood are found in limbic structures, and those mediating endocrine effects are located in the hypothalamus. Opiate receptors are also found in more peripheral sites of the nervous system, such as the myenteric plexuses of the bowel, in peripheral nerves in areas of inflammation, and in smooth muscle sphincters, such as those of the bladder or bile ducts.

Opioids can be classified as agonists or antagonists according to their effects on each of the types of opiate receptors. Agonist opioids bind to receptors and activate them to produce analgesia and other wanted and unwanted effects. Opioid antagonists such as naloxone bind to receptors but do not activate them. They compete with agonist drugs for binding sites and block the effects of agonists, and are therefore useful in reversing respiratory depression in patients who have taken an overdose of an agonist opioid such as morphine. None of the exogenous opioids has specificity for only one receptor, and that is why the analgesia is often associated with unwanted or adverse effects.

Agonist-antagonist drugs have a variety of both agonist and antagonist effects at opiate receptors. The analgesic effects of these drugs have ceilings (higher dosages have no extra benefits), and the drugs may cause withdrawal when administered to patients taking pure agonists. The action of partial agonist drugs such as buprenorphine and nalbuphine is not well understood, and their clinical usefulness is limited.

■ **Pharmacokinetics.** Opioids are absorbed relatively well from the gastrointestinal tract. However, first-pass metabolism in the liver accounts for the reduced bioavailability of oral opioids compared with that of parenteral opioids.

Opioids disperse widely in the body and cross the blood-brain barrier, although some opioids like morphine may cross more slowly.

Opioids are metabolized in the liver to glucuronides, which are excreted primarily in the urine but also in the bile. Morphine-6-glucuronide is an active metabolite producing analgesia and other CNS effects. This metabolite is probably responsible for a significant amount of analgesic effect observed with long-term morphine administration. Morphine-3-glucuronide is not an analgesic, but may be an active mediator of opioid adverse effects. Other opioids have metabolites but their role in analgesia and in producing side effects is not clear. Renal dysfunction results in decreased clearance of these metabolites and, therefore, may cause increased analgesic effects as well as increased toxic effects. Hepatic dysfunction, until very severe, does not seem to have the same effect. There is no clear evidence yet for choosing one opioid over another on the basis of activity of metabolites alone, except possibly in renal failure or hepatic failure. All strong opioids or their metabolites may accumulate in the face of renal or hepatic failure. Since there is limited information at the moment, patients with such conditions need to be monitored carefully and dosages lowered if side effects such as severe myoclonus develop.

Duration of action is a function of protein-binding, distribution in the cerebrospinal fluid and metabolism. See Table 5.

- **Physical dependence and tolerance.** All patients chronically taking morphine and other opioids for pain control can exhibit some tolerance and require upward adjustments of dosage, but the effect is minimal and does not require ever-increasing dosages. Increases in opioid dose requirement are usually related to disease progression.[1] Physical dependence also occurs, so patients on opioids for long periods may exhibit some withdrawal symptoms if the drug is suddenly stopped or if antagonist drugs are given purposely or inadvertently. *Addiction, which differs from physical dependence or tolerance, is very rare in patients who take opioids for chronic severe cancer pain.*

- **Endogenous opioids.** Three groups of endogenous opioids—enkephalins, endorphins and dynorphin—act at opiate receptor sites and are the subject of intense research, but their roles and significance are not yet entirely clear.

Table 5: Opioid Analgesics

The following dosage equivalents of immediate-release opioids to morphine 10 mg parenteral were initially based mainly on single-dose studies. They are guidelines only in patients requiring chronic administration. See text for further information.

Drug	Parenteral Dose	Dose p.o.	Immediate-Release Dose Frequency[*]
Recommended			
Codeine	120 mg	180 to 240 mg	q3 to 4h
Oxycodone	15 mg	10 to 15 mg	q3 to 4h
Fentanyl (transdermal)	Not applicable	25 µg/hr	Every 3 days
Heroin[†]	6 mg	12 to 20 mg	q3 to 4h
Hydromorphone[‡]	2 mg	4 to 6 mg	q3 to 4h
Methadone[§,‖]			
Morphine	10 mg	20 to 30 mg	q3 to 4h
Not Recommended			
Anileridine	25 mg	75 to 100 mg	q2 to 3h
Butorphanol[¶]	2 mg	Not applicable	q3 to 4h
Levorphanol	2 mg	4 mg	q6h
Meperidine	75 mg	200 to 300 mg	q2 to 3h
Nalbuphine[‡]	10 mg	Not applicable	q3 to 6h
Oxymorphone	1.5 mg	5 mg (p.r.)[**]	q4h
Pentazocine[¶]	60 mg	180 mg	q3 to 4h

* generally the shorter frequency is appropriate with the s.c. dose only

† not available in Canada for oral use

‡ can be used intravenously or subcutaneously

§ recommended only if physician familiar with the special features of this drug, and as a second-line opioid only under the supervision of experts in pain management and palliative care

‖ extremely variable equianalgesic dose; patients should undergo individualized titration starting at equivalent to 1/10 of the morphine dose

¶ agonist-antagonist drugs

** per rectum

Weak Opioid Analgesics

When a non-opioid analgesic fails to control mild to moderate pain, a weak opioid analgesic may be added to the regimen. Although weak opioids include agonist drugs—codeine, oxycodone combination products, and dextropropoxyphene—and the agonist-antagonist drug pentazocine, the choice of useful weak opioids is limited to two pure agonist drugs: codeine and oxycodone/acetaminophen or oxycodone/ASA combination drugs. Dextropropoxyphene probably has little role to play since it is controversial whether it has any action over and above placebo. Pentazocine has unacceptably high psychotomimetic effects and oral forms are absorbed poorly. The classification of oxycodone combination drugs as weak analgesics is based upon the reasoning described below.

■ **Codeine.** Codeine, the "gold standard" for the weak opioids, is well absorbed both orally and subcutaneously. It is partly converted to morphine in the body, which contributes to its effects. Codeine is most widely used in combination with acetaminophen or ASA. The extra analgesic effect provided by these drug combinations is usually seen only when at least 60 mg of codeine has been added. Plain codeine tablets or elixir can be added to increase codeine dosage; however, in our clinical experience it is rarely useful to exceed 120 mg of codeine orally every 4 hours (720 mg/day). If more codeine seems to be needed for better pain control, it is best to change to morphine or another more potent opioid. Patients who take more than 2 tablets of combination products every 4 hours should be monitored for adverse effects of ASA or acetaminophen. Codeine is available in a controlled-release formulation (see Chapter 7, p. 50) that can avoid ceiling doses of non-opioid agents that are part of combination products. See Table 6 for formulations and recommended dosage.

Table 6: Codeine Formulations and Recommended Dosage

FORMULATIONS	DOSAGE
Oral	
Plain tablets 30, 60 mg	60 to 120 mg q4h
Elixir/syrup 3 to 5 mg/mL	60 to 120 mg q4h
Acetaminophen 325 mg with codeine 30 mg or 60 mg	2 to 3 tablets q4h*
ASA 325 mg with codeine 30 mg or 60 mg	2 to 3 tablets q4h*
Controlled-release tablets 50, 100, 150, 200 mg	100 to 300 mg q12h
Parenteral	60 to 180 mg q3 to 4h

* at maximum dosage for long-term use, renal and hepatic function should be monitored

■ Oxycodone. When prescribed in combination with ASA or acetaminophen, oxycodone may be classed as a weak opioid, but when used alone and appropriately titrated, it is a strong opioid. The pharmacologic characteristics of oxycodone are listed on pages 46-47. However, when dispensed in fixed combination with non-opioid drugs, maximum dosage is determined by the possible toxicity of the non-opioid agents, not by the amount of oxycodone. Oxycodone alone is available in immediate- and controlled-release formulations that can avoid ceiling doses of non-opioid agents that are part of combination products. See Table 7 for oxycodone combination formulations and recommended dosage.

Table 7: Oxycodone Combination Formulations and Recommended Dosage

FORMULATIONS	DOSAGE
Oral	
Acetaminophen 325 mg with oxycodone 5 mg	2 to 3 tablets q4h*
ASA 325 mg with oxycodone 5 mg	2 to 3 tablets q4h*

* at maximum dosage for long-term use, renal and hepatic function should be monitored

- **Pentazocine.** *Pentazocine is not recommended for use in cancer pain.* Classification of pentazocine as a weak opioid is related to its limited bioavailability, which requires at least 3 or 4 times the usual parenteral dose of 60 mg. But the available oral preparations do not reflect that fact. The incidence of psychotomimetic side effects is much higher than with other agents. The antagonist properties of pentazocine also limit its use in combination with other opioids.

- **Dextropropoxyphene.** *Dextropropoxyphene is not recommended for use in cancer pain.* It is a weak opioid that has not been shown to have much activity above placebo.

Strong Opioids

Strong opioids are the analgesics of choice when cancer pain is moderate or severe. Morphine is the parent and the "gold standard" of this group. As with weak opioids, strong opioids are usually agonist or agonist-antagonist in action. Agonist-antagonist strong opioids such as nalbuphine and butorphanol are not recommended because they offer little advantage and considerable disadvantage due to their antagonist activity.

The strong opioids include the drugs morphine, hydromorphone, heroin, oxycodone, methadone, fentanyl, levorphanol, oxymorphone, meperidine and anileridine.

- **Morphine.** Morphine is a natural compound and is the major active component of opium. When administered orally, it is well absorbed and, with regular dosing, it is about one-half as potent as it is by the parenteral route. The usual duration of action of immediate-release oral morphine is about 4 hours; for parenteral morphine it is about 3 to 4 hours (Table 8). Morphine sulfate has limited solubility in water (about 65 mg/mL), which limits its concentration in parenteral preparations.

Table 8: Morphine Formulations

FORMULATION	AVAILABLE DOSAGE FORMS
Oral	Liquid 1, 5, 10, 20, 50 mg/mL
	Immediate-release tablets 5, 10, 15, 20, 25, 30, 50, 60 mg
	Controlled-release tablets or capsules 10, 15, 30, 60, 100, 200 mg*
Rectal	Immediate-release suppositories 5, 10, 20, 30 mg
	Controlled-release suppositories 30, 60, 100, 200 mg*
Parenteral	Morphine sulfate 10, 15, 20, 25, 50 mg/mL

*see section on controlled-release products, pp. 57-59

Morphine is principally metabolized in the liver and yet-to-be identified extrahepatic sites. The metabolite morphine-6-glucuronide exerts a potent analgesic effect. Other metabolites—morphine-3-glucuronide and normorphine—have no analgesic effects. The other effects of all these metabolites have been investigated with conflicting results in human and animal models. They may account for some of the toxicity that can be seen in some patients with long-term administration of morphine. The dosage forms of morphine are described in Table 8. For recommended dosages of strong opioids see the section on dosage (pp. 53-56).

■ **Hydromorphone.** Hydromorphone is a semi-synthetic agent that is about 5 times more potent than morphine; however, in equianalgesic doses it is no more effective in relieving pain. It is well absorbed orally, and its oral-to-parenteral ratio is 2:1. The major metabolite, hydromorphone-3-glucuronide, is not analgesic but might have other effects that, as yet, have not been conclusively documented in humans. Case reports of hydromorphone toxicity and accumulation of hydromorphone-3-glucuronide in renal failure have appeared in the literature.[2,3] The profile of adverse effects is the same as for morphine. When high parenteral doses of analgesic are required, hydromorphone might have an important advantage over morphine sulfate because it is more soluble (up to 300 mg/mL); thus, the injection volume can be much lower. Recently, a controlled-release formulation has been made available. See Table 9 for formulations.

Table 9: Hydromorphone Formulations

FORMULATIONS	AVAILABLE DOSAGE FORMS
Oral	Liquid 1 mg/mL
	Immediate-release tablets 1, 2, 4, 8 mg
	Controlled-release capsules 3, 6, 12, 24 mg*
Rectal	Immediate-release suppositories 3 mg
Parenteral	Prepared solutions 1, 2, 10, 20, 50 mg/mL
	Powder for reconstitution

* see section on controlled-release products, pp. 57-59

- **Heroin.** In Canada, heroin (diacetylmorphine) for parenteral administration is available for limited use in hospitals. It is about 1.5 to 2 times more potent than morphine, but it is no more effective in equianalgesic doses. There is no scientific evidence or even consistent descriptive evidence to support the myth that heroin provides euphoria for patients. It is more soluble than morphine sulfate or hydromorphone (up to 600 mg/mL); therefore, it may be used to make up very concentrated solutions for patients who require large parenteral doses of strong opioids. However, when the issue of potency is considered along with solubility, hydromorphone, not heroin, is in our clinical experience the parenteral drug of choice if small injection volumes are required.

- **Oxycodone.** Oxycodone has pharmacokinetics similar to those of morphine. Its oral bioavailability is greater than that of morphine and its oral to parenteral ratio is 1:2. When oxycodone is given orally, its relative analgesic potency, compared with morphine, is 2:1. Its side effect profile is the same as morphine. Similar to other opioids, oxycodone metabolites may have some pharmacologic activity but are not considered to contribute significantly to the analgesic effect.

Table 10: Plain Oxycodone Formulations

Formulation	Available Dosage Forms
Oral	Immediate-release tablets 5, 10 mg
Oral	Controlled-release tablets 10, 20, 40, 80 mg*
Rectal	Immediate-release suppositories 10, 20 mg

*see section on controlled-release products, pp. 57-59

■ **Methadone.** The major theoretical advantage of methadone is its longer duration of analgesic action. It has excellent bioavailability by the oral and rectal routes. Its half-life is variable (6 to 20 hr; mean: 15 hr) but this unfortunately increases unpredictably with repeated dosing. The resultant accumulation can expose patients to sudden severe toxicity. In Canada, the use of methadone requires a special licence, and the drug is difficult to obtain. It may be used in the rare patient who is truly allergic to morphine and it may have a role to play in opioid rotation ("High-Dose Opioids" section, p. 60). *Methadone is generally recommended as a second-line opioid only under the supervision of experts in pain management and palliative care.*

■ **Fentanyl.** Fentanyl and related drugs are strong, very short-acting synthetic opioids that have been used in the past mainly during general anesthesia or for epidural administration. The transdermal delivery route has been shown to be reliable and effective.[4,5] Family physicians should have skill in using opioids such as morphine before using fentanyl patches because of the complex pharmacokinetics of the transdermal delivery system (see Chapter 10, p. 73).

- **Levorphanol.** Levorphanol is a synthetic opioid of high potency. It has a longer duration of action than morphine—around 6 hours. It also has a long half-life and can accumulate in patients, producing toxicity. *Levorphanol has no distinct advantages, and because of its tendency to accumulate, it is not recommended for general use in patients with chronic cancer pain. Its use should be carefully supervised by experts in the handling of opioid drugs.*

- **Oxymorphone.** Oxymorphone has no advantages over morphine and is available in Canada only as a single-strength rectal suppository. *Because of this limited dosage and route flexibility, oxymorphone is not recommended for patients with chronic cancer pain.*

- **Meperidine.** Meperidine is usually classed as a potent opioid. It has little role to play in the management of chronic pain in cancer patients but might be a drug of choice for acute pain. It has a short duration of action (1 to 3 hr). It is poorly absorbed orally, with an oral-to-parenteral ratio of 4:1. Normeperidine, a metabolite of meperidine, is not an active analgesic metabolite but can lead to neurologic side effects including seizures. *Meperidine is not recommended for use in chronic cancer pain.*

- **Anileridine.** Anileridine is from the same family of drugs as meperidine; therefore, it shares some of the same features, particularly the short duration of action when taken orally. It is available in fixed dosage tablets only, which limits its flexibility in titrating dosage. *Because it offers no advantages over morphine, it is not recommended that anileridine be used routinely in chronic cancer pain.*

References

1. Collin E, Poulin P, Guuvain-Piquard A et al. Is disease progression the major factor in morphine "tolerance" in cancer pain treatment? *Pain* 1993; 55: 319- 26.

2. Fainsinger R, Schoeller T, Boiskin M, Bruera E. Palliative care round: Cognitive failure and coma after renal failure in a patient receiving captopril and hydromorphone. *J Palliative Care* 1993; 9:53-5.

3. Babul N, Darke AC, Hagen N. Hydromorphone metabolite accumulation in renal failure. *J Pain Sympt Manage* 1995; 10:184-6.

4. Mosser KH. Transdermal fentanyl in cancer pain. *Am Fam Phys* 1992; 45:2289-94.

5. Donner B, Zenz M. Transdermal fentanyl: a new step on the therapeutic ladder. *Anti-Cancer Drugs* 1995; 6(Suppl. 3):39-43.

7 *Effective Use of Opioids*

Using Opioids More Effectively

The following guidelines should be remembered.

1. **Understand the pharmacology of the clinically-useful opioids.** The successful use of opioids depends critically on a clear understanding of their effects, positive and adverse (see Chapter 9, p. 63).

2. **Educate the patient, family and other service providers about opioids.** Before ordering any opioid, what is being done must be explained to the patient, family and other service providers. It is essential to discuss in detail the pain-control objectives, the expected effects, the potential adverse effects and how they will be treated, the dosage regimen, the use of breakthrough medication, the use of adjuncts and the responsibilities for monitoring. It is important also to take time to explore the ever-present concerns including fears of addiction and of adverse effects; and to reassure patient and family.

3. **Always provide a breakthrough dose** (pp. 55-56). The supplemental breakthrough dose is essential to handle the common phenomenon of increased pain that "breaks through" the baseline level because it is becoming less well-controlled, or not controlled at all, or it peaks at particular times for whatever reason. Generally, the frequency of administration of breakthrough doses should be specified as at least hourly. The patient should be instructed to take this extra medication and record the number of extra doses taken and why. This medication record should be reviewed routinely by caregivers and adjustments in the regular dose made if more than two or three breakthrough doses are required between regular doses in a 24-hour period. In institutional settings, nurses must be aware of the need to deliver breakthrough medication quickly.

Figure 5

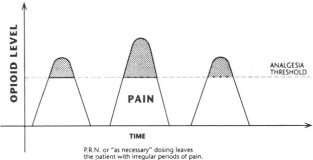

P.R.N. or "as necessary" dosing leaves
the patient with irregular periods of pain.

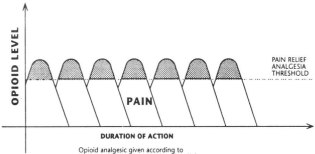

Opioid analgesic given according to
duration of action to maintain pain relief.

Some institutions have policies where breakthrough medicine can be left at the patient's bedside. This is also an excellent idea at home. Current practice calls for the breakthrough medication to be the immediate-release formulation of the same strong opioid. There is currently no established way of supplementing transdermal fentanyl with oral fentanyl so another immediate-release strong opioid should be used.

4. **Give opioids orally unless contraindicated.** Oral opioids can be effective even when the pain is severe. The oral route is often mistakenly thought to be inefficient and

impractical, frequently because adverse effects such as nausea and vomiting have not been managed appropriately.

5. **Give opioids regularly according to the duration of their analgesic effect.** Providing analgesics "as necessary" leaves the patient open to periods of pain interspersed with periods of relief. In institutions, this regimen can also leave to busy caregivers the task of interpreting the patient's need for pain medication and when to give it. Regular administration of opioids prevents pain and allows relatively smooth pain control.

6. **Anticipate and prevent adverse effects.** The common adverse effects of opioids are predictable and frequent. The clinician must anticipate these when prescribing an opioid and take a preventive approach right from the beginning. Treatment of the common adverse effects is described in Chapter 9 (p. 63).

7. **Determine an appropriate starting dose.** There is no exact way to determine how much of a strong opioid a patient will need to control pain. An individualized approach is required. However, there are some general guidelines that can be followed. These are described in detail on pages 53-56.

8. **There is no upper limit to opioid dosage.** Many patients will be controlled with a total daily dose of 360 mg of morphine or less, or equivalent dose of another opioid. However, the dose should be increased until either pain control is achieved or adverse effects become intolerable.

9. **Do not mix opioid drugs.** Combinations of agonist and agonist-antagonist drugs, or weak and strong opioids, should be avoided (see Chapter 6, pp. 38-39).

10. **Always consider using non-opioid analgesics along with strong opioids.** The different actions of those drugs might be complementary in relieving pain, especially bone pain.

11. Remember that some types of pain may not be fully responsive to opioid analgesics. See Chapter 9, pp. 79-84.

12. Always remember the concept of total pain. Opioids are just one part of the solution of a patient's pain problems. All the other areas described in the concept of total pain (pp. 11-12) must be addressed.

Guidelines for Determining the Initial Dosage of Strong Opioids

1. **Drug selection.** Unless there are overwhelming contraindications, one should start with morphine or hydromorphone.

2. **Dosage form.** In most cases, one should start with immediate-release forms in the most flexible dosage form possible to make dosage titration easier. Liquid preparations may provide greater flexibility, but immediate-release tablets can also be used. If liquid preparations are used, one must ensure that the dose is measured accurately with special measuring devices or syringes. Also, the most concentrated liquid form feasible should be used as smaller volumes are much better tolerated, especially in patients who have difficulty with taste or appearance of liquid medication. However, patients may prefer to take tablets of immediate-release preparations.

Table 11: Initial Doses of Strong Opioids

Drug	Immediate-Release Dosage
First-Line	
Morphine	10 to 20 mg q4h
Hydromorphone	3 to 6 mg q4h
Other Choices	
Fentanyl transdermal*	25 µg/hr patch every 2 to 3 days

*see page 77 for situations where fentanyl may be first choice

3. **The opioid-naive patient.** In the patient who has received little or no strong opioid in the last 24 to 48 hours, the usual starting dose should be equivalent to 10 to 20 mg morphine q4h.

4. **Conversion to oral medication.** In patients who have received frequent, strong parenteral opioids within the last 24 hours, one should add up the total dose given in a 24-hour period. If pain control was fair or adequate at that dosage level, one may divide that total daily amount by 6 and then double the result to obtain a reasonable 4-hourly starting dose of oral immediate-release strong opioid. One can then easily multiply that result by 3 to determine the 12-hourly dose of controlled-release preparations.

   For example, if the patient had received 120 mg of morphine parenterally in the previous 24 hours and had adequate pain control, the appropriate 4-hourly oral dose would be calculated as follows:

   120/6 x 2 = 40 mg q4h of oral immediate-release morphine converted to controlled-release morphine by multiplying by 3 for a total of 120 mg q12h.

   If pain was poorly controlled, this method could be used, but one would increase the dose of immediate-release morphine by 25 to 50 percent. Using the example above in a patient with poorly controlled pain, the 4-hourly dose would be 40 x 1.5 = 60 mg q4h of immediate-release morphine.

   For the patient with poorly controlled pain, converting to controlled-release preparations is not recommended until adequate analgesia has been achieved.

5. **Severe pain.** In patients with very severe or overwhelming pain, consider regular parenteral dosing (p. 74) or the use of constant subcutaneous infusion (pp. 74-75) for the first 24 to 48 hours.

6. **Dose titration.** Dose titration is one of the keys to success in using opioids effectively, since requirements will be individual to each patient. The aim is to find the optimum

dose of regularly-administered opioid that will maintain the patient as free of pain as possible. Dose adjustments should be determined by the patient's response. The dose should be changed every 16 to 24 hours until pain is controlled. Instructions should be left with patient and family about the next step for an increase in the regular dose, or the physician contact them at the appropriate interval.

- When initiating opioids, the dose should be increased by 15 to 25 percent every 24 hours unless there are uncontrolled adverse effects.

- In institutions, orders for the opioid should be written using a range of doses so that the nurses can increase the dose at their discretion (e.g., 10 to 20 mg morphine q4h p.o.).

- Dose increases should vary according to the regular dose and should take into account the number of breakthrough doses.

- If more than two or three breakthrough doses are required regularly between the established dose over a 24-hour period, the total amount of breakthrough medication given should be added to the 24-hour total and the dose of the immediate-release or controlled-release opioid recalculated.

7. **Special cases.** Altering dosage should be considered in special situations.

- In renal failure, reduced dosage and longer dosage intervals should in general be used; one should monitor frequently for toxicity.

- At the end of life when fluid intake and renal output decrease, altering dosage should be considered.

- In the very frail elderly, smaller starting doses should be used (e.g., 2 to 5 mg morphine equivalents q4h).

- In patients with a history of severe adverse effects from opioids, one should start with smaller doses, sometimes very small doses.

8. **Breakthrough dose.** The breakthrough dose should vary and increase with increments of the regular opioid dose. *A general formula to apply is that the breakthrough dose should be one-third to one-half of the regular q4h dose or approximately one-fifth of the scheduled q12h dose of controlled-release preparations.*

9. **Stable dose.** When a stable dose has been reached, one should consider switching to controlled-release preparations to simplify drug administration regimens for the patient and family.

Table 12: Summary Table of Opioids: Recommendations

WEAK OPIOIDS/AGONIST DRUGS	
Recommended	*Not Recommended*
Codeine	Dextropropoxyphene
Oxycodone combination products	
STRONG OPIOIDS/AGONIST DRUGS	
Recommended	*Not Recommended*
Morphine	Anileridine
Hydromorphone	Levorphanol
Fentanyl (transdermal)	Meperidine
Oxycodone	Oxymorphone
Methadone*	
STRONG OPIOIDS/AGONIST-ANTAGONIST DRUGS	
	Not Recommended
	Butorphanol
	Nalbuphine
	Pentazocine

*recommended only if physician familiar with the special features of this drug, and as a second-line opioid only under the supervision of experts in pain management and palliative care

Oral Controlled-Release Opioid Preparations

The controlled-release preparations[1-4] have simplified the long-term administration of opioids because they contain opioids within different types of matrices that dissolve slowly to release the opioid drug gradually and fairly consistently in the intestines.

Several oral formulations are available: codeine, hydromorphone, morphine and oxycodone. It should be explained carefully to the patient, family and nurses that controlled-release tablets cannot be broken (except for the codeine tablets and the 200 mg morphine tablet, which can be split in half) or crushed because this will increase the release of drug substantially and possibly lead to toxicity. Similarly, although pellet formulations can be opened, the pellets must not be chewed or crushed in any way.

Controlled-release preparations of opioids are not bioequivalent and should not be considered interchangeable since they all have different matrices and different drug-release characteristics.

The spectrum of adverse effects of controlled-release preparations is no different from those of the immediate-release preparations. However, in patients who have adverse effects related to the peak of absorption of immediate-release opioids, the longer-acting drugs may cause fewer or less severe adverse effects.

- **Absorption.** There are two types of oral controlled-release analgesic preparations: one given every 12 hours and one given every 24 hours. The peak absorption of controlled-release preparations given every 12 hours is usually around 3 to 4 hours, although this may vary. The duration of analgesic effect is up to 12 hours. If the patient's pain is breaking through at 10 to 12 hours, then the 12-hour dosage should be increased appropriately. If good pain control is not achieved with an appropriate dosage increase or side effects are associated with the peak morphine concentration, patients may benefit from 8-hourly administration. Certainly, controlled-release preparations should not be given any more frequently than every 8 hours. The once-daily controlled-release preparation peak absorption is around 8 hours. Where judged necessary, it may be administered more frequently than 24 hours, but no more often than q12h. These controlled-release preparations should probably not be used in patients with significantly shortened bowel (e.g., ileostomy), rapid intestinal transit (e.g., diarrhea) or in patients with chronic nausea and vomiting.

- **Dosage.** Once a stable dose of opioid has been reached using the immediate-release preparations, the patient can generally be switched to the oral controlled-release preparations. The dose of controlled-release opioid is determined by dividing the total daily dose of immediate-release opioid by 2 to get the q12h dose or by 3 to get the q8h dose.

- **Breakthrough medication** *should always be in the form of oral immediate-release tablets or liquid of the same opioid.* The breakthrough dose can be one-fifth of the scheduled 12-hourly dose. If frequent breakthrough doses are required, then the total daily dose of controlled-release medication should be increased by at least the breakthrough amount in a 24-hour period.

Table 13: Oral Controlled-Release Preparations

DRUG	TRADE NAME	DOSAGES
Morphine	MS Contin®	15, 30, 60, 100, 200 mg tablets
	M-Eslon®	10, 15, 30, 60, 100, 200 mg capsules
	MOS-SR™	30, 60 mg tablets
	Oramorph SR™	30, 60, 100 mg tablets
Hydromorphone	Hydromorph Contin®	3, 6, 12, 24 mg capsules
Codeine	Codeine Contin®	50, 100, 150, 200 mg tablets
Oxycodone	OxyContin®	10, 20, 40, 80 mg tablets
*Morphine**	Kadian®	20, 50, 100 mg capsules

* once-daily dosing

References

1. Walsh TD. A controlled study of MS-tablets for chronic pain in advanced cancer. In Wilkes E, Levy J (eds), *Advances in Morphine Therapy*. Royal Society of Medicine. International Congress and Symposium Series. London 1981; 58:99-102.

2. Hays H, Hagen N, Thirlwell M et al. Comparative clinical efficacy and safety of immediate-release and controlled-release hydromorphone for chronic severe cancer pain. *Cancer* 1994; 74:1808-16.

3. Chary S, Goughnour BR, Moulin DE et al. The dose-response relationship of controlled-release codeine (Codeine Contin) in chronic cancer pain. *J Pain Sympt Manage* 1994; 9:363-71.

4. Dhaliwal HS, Sloan P, Arkinstall W et al. Randomized evaluation of controlled-release codeine and placebo in chronic cancer pain. *J Pain Sympt Manage* 1995; 10:612-23.

8 Special Issues in Using Opioids

High-Dose Opioids

About 20 percent of cancer patients with chronic severe pain will require more than an equivalent of 600 mg of morphine daily. For many physicians this is a formidable psychologic barrier, but fears about high-dose opioids are groundless. There is, in fact, no fixed upper limit to strong opioid dosage. Higher doses are not an absolute indication of tolerance or addiction; they are usually an indication of pain severity, opioid-resistant pain, anxiety and/or other metabolic factors affecting drug kinetics. Higher doses may be associated with increasing adverse effects, particularly neurotoxic effects such as hallucinations and myoclonus. Adverse effects should be treated aggressively, yet ongoing rotation among opioid analgesics may be necessary to manage uncontrolled side effects in some patients effectively.

Opioids in the Elderly

The elderly are often more sensitive to effects of all types of medications. The reasons for this are complex but include changes in drug metabolism, changes in protein binding, increased numbers of medications prescribed enhancing the possibility of drug interactions and other physiologic changes associated with aging.

Analgesics can be used in most elderly patients in the same fashion as described previously. However, a number of issues need to be considered.

- In the frail elderly, starting doses may need to be lowered and titration may be a little more prolonged than usual.
- Sedation is more common in the elderly.

- Elderly patients with some pre-existing cognitive problems may be more sensitive to the psychotomimetic effects of opioids. Pain problems in such patients may require very low doses in initiating therapy and more gradual titration.

- Elderly patients with some pre-existing cognitive problems need to be monitored more carefully in regard to medication compliance. Special medication reminder-aids such as Dosett™ containers (i.e., dispensing boxes with partitions to store different pills) may be needed to simplify medication administration.

- Elderly patients often have decreased renal function and need to be monitored more carefully for toxicity due to reduced elimination of metabolites.

Opioids at the End of Life

In most cases, opioids should be continued unabated until the end of a patient's life. However, some circumstances may indicate a need to modify opioid dosing.

- As renal clearance decreases secondary to reduced fluid intake and dehydration, metabolites may build up and produce toxicity. Opioid dosage may need to be decreased and/or the frequency changed to reflect prolonged effects. Immediate-release preparations are probably preferred in this situation.

- In the patient with a decreasing level of consciousness, the perception of pain may diminish and the dosage of opioid can be decreased if signs of toxicity such as myoclonus are evident.

- In the patient in deep coma, the continuation of opioids is controversial. Pain is subjective and requires conscious appreciation, which is lacking in patients in deep coma. Opioids may be stopped only if the patient is monitored carefully for any signs of pain.

Low-Dose Opioids

A small number of patients may exhibit considerable sensitivity to the effects of strong opioids. These patients tell a story of intractable side effects such as extreme sedation with the usual starting doses of strong opioids. The approach in these patients should involve initiating doses of opioids that are very low (e.g., 1 mg morphine or 0.25 mg of hydromorphone every 4 hours or less with slow titration upwards). Often doses remain quite small with good pain control.

9 *Adverse Effects of Opioids*

Pain control probably would be much easier, and more progress would have been made much earlier in the techniques of pain control if opioids did not have frequent and significant adverse effects. Nevertheless, the major adverse effects of opioid drugs are mostly transient, predictable, rarely very serious and usually relatively easy to manage.

Controlling Adverse Effects

The basic principles listed below need to be followed in managing the common adverse effects of opioids:

- understanding the pharmacology of opioids;
- taking a good history of the adverse reaction;
- remembering that symptoms that are the same as the common adverse effects of opioids (e.g., nausea, sedation, etc.) might not be due to the opioid alone or to the opioid at all;
- using a physiologic and preventive approach to managing adverse effects of opioids;
- giving medication for adverse effects orally and regularly;
- remembering that medications for adverse effects will have adverse effects themselves; therefore, one should use as little as necessary and monitor the patient frequently;
- being flexible;
- always educating patient and family about these unwanted but common effects of opioids.

Nausea and Vomiting

Nausea and vomiting occur in 50 to 70 percent of patients exposed to opioids; therefore, the best approach is to prescribe an antiemetic along with the opioid, at least for the first few days.

Morphine and other opioids cause nausea by three direct mechanisms: primarily, by direct stimulation of the chemoreceptor trigger zone; relatively commonly, by decreased stomach and bowel motility; infrequently, by vestibular stimulation.

There are many potential causes of nausea in cancer patients, and they may need to be ruled out before assuming the nausea is due to the opioid.

Other causes of nausea in cancer patients include:

- constipation;
- other medications (e.g., NSAIDs, amitriptyline, carbamazepine, etc.);
- bowel obstruction;
- metabolic disturbances, such as renal failure and hypercalcemia;
- hepatomegaly;
- invasion of celiac plexus by tumor;
- anxiety;
- dislike of liquid medication;
- effects of chemotherapy or radiotherapy;
- raised intracranial pressure.

Management of Opioid-Induced Nausea

The following guidelines should be used in managing opioid-induced nausea.

- **Prescribe an antiemetic** along with the strong opioids, unless there is a good reason to suspect the patient will not have nausea (e.g., previous exposure to strong opioids has not produced nausea). Many patients will require p.r.n. doses of antiemetics. Some patients with chronic nausea will require round-the-clock dosing.

- **Select an appropriate antiemetic** according to a physiologic approach:

  - for most patients the first-line drugs include those that affect the chemoreceptor trigger zone (Table 14);

- if stomach motility seems to be an issue (patient feels full all the time) or if a first-line drug is not working, try adding motility agents (Table 15).

Table 14: Suggested Antiemetics for Opioid-Induced Nausea

DRUG	DOSAGE	COMMENTS
First-Line Agent		
Haloperidol	0.5 to 5 mg s.c. or p.o. once daily to t.i.d.	Adverse effects rare at low dose; usual dose is less than 2 mg daily
Secondary Drug		
Prochlorperazine	5 to 10 mg i.m., p.r., or p.o. every 6 hours	Dystonic effects and sedation may occur
Other Drugs		
Chlorpromazine	25 to 50 mg i.m. or p.o. every 6 hours	Dystonic effects and sedation may occur
Dimenhydrinate	25 to 50 mg i.m. or p.o. 4 to 6 hours	Especially if vertigo present Sedation may occur
Metoclopramide	5 to 20 mg q.i.d.	Adverse effects can include extrapyramidal symptoms; available soon in controlled-release formulation

Table 15: Motility Agents

DRUG	DOSAGE	COMMENTS
Domperidone	10 to 40 mg q.i.d.	Not necessary to give before meals
Cisapride	5 to 20 mg q.i.d.	May cause diarrhea
Metoclopramide	5 to 20 mg q.i.d.	Adverse effects can include extrapyramidal symptoms; available soon in controlled-release formulation

- **Search out other causes of nausea,** especially constipation and other medications, and correct as necessary.

- **Monitor the patient** and reassess the need for antiemetics every few days; many patients will not need continuing doses of antiemetics unless the dose is rapidly increased again.

- **Switch to another strong opioid** or try a different route of administration of opioid if nausea remains a major problem after 2 to 3 days and is most likely due to the opioid, other causes having been ruled out.

- **Prescribe dexamethasone,** 16 to 24 mg daily for 3 to 5 days, which may be effective in patients with severe, intractable and very distressing nausea, and in vomiting where the cause is unknown and where there are no major contraindications to steroid use. The mechanism of action is not known and not well documented by research data.

Constipation

Constipation is almost universal in patients taking opioids and can cause significant suffering and increase pain. Constipation results from opioid interference with bowel motility at the level of the myenteric plexus, which causes poor propulsion of intestinal contents. It is probably best to be aggressive and prescribe a bowel regimen routinely with every opioid. The patient needs to be monitored daily and carefully for constipation.

Other causes of constipation in these patients include:

- a diet deficient in fibre and other natural laxative elements;
- inactivity;
- severe weakness;
- anxiety about using the bedpan or commode;
- other medications such as amitriptyline or NSAIDs;
- bowel obstruction;
- a history of major problems with constipation;

- metabolic disturbances;
- dehydration;
- lack of privacy.

Management of Constipation

The following guidelines should be used in managing constipation.

- **Monitor patients well.** This might involve having the patient or family keep some sort of record.

- **Do a rectal exam.** Patients with a severe impaction might require instillation of mineral oil and subsequent manual disimpaction; patients with an empty but ballooned-out rectum may have a higher obstruction from a fecal mass, and will require high enemas to clear the constipation.

- **Do a flat x-ray of the abdomen.** If the diagnosis is unclear, this may be the only way to find out if the patient has severe constipation.

- **Correct the diet,** if possible. In relatively well patients this is usually helpful; however, patients with advanced cancer and those with significant anorexia are not likely to take foods with much fibre or be able to take fibre supplements. Therefore, trying to increase dietary fibre should not be a major goal in many patients. Increased fluid intake may be helpful.

- **Prescribe regular doses of laxatives orally.** Usually a combination of a softener and a stimulant is required. Large doses of laxatives are often needed (Table 16, p. 68).

- **Use glycerin or bisacodyl suppositories** if oral agents are ineffective after 3 days.

- **Use a phosphate or soapsuds saline enema** if suppositories are ineffective; if the obstruction is higher up, then an oil-retention enema can be used followed hours later by a soapsuds or saline enema. Enema technique is important and high instillation of oil and other liquids is required.

Table 16: **Laxative Drugs**

LAXATIVE TYPE	DOSAGE	COMMENTS
Stool Softeners		
Docusate sodium capsules	100 to 200 mg b.i.d.	Rarely worth going above 4 capsules daily
Docusate sodium liquid	10 to 30 mL b.i.d.	Bad taste
Docusate calcium capsules	240 to 480 mg b.i.d.	
Stimulant Laxatives		
Senna tablets 8.6 mg	2 to 6 tablets b.i.d.	Can cause cramping
Senna syrup	10 to 30 mL b.i.d.	
Senna suppository 30 mg	1 p.r. every 2 to 3 days	
Bisacodyl 5 mg tablets	2 to 6 tablets b.i.d.	Can cause cramping
Bisacodyl suppository 10 mg	1 p.r. every 2 to 3 days	
Glycerin suppository	1 p.r. every 2 to 3 days	
Stimulants and Softeners		
Senna + docusate sodium	2 to 6 tablets b.i.d.	
Osmotic Agents		
Lactulose	15 to 60 mL b.i.d.	Taste and texture may be poorly tolerated
Magnesium citrate	250 mL bottle	For severe constipation
Saline Cathartics		
Milk of magnesia	30 to 60 mL b.i.d.	

Sedation or Drowsiness

Some minor degree of sedation is experienced by most patients when they first begin to take opioids, especially strong opioids. It does not require any treatment except reassurance to the patient and family that the effect will usually clear in a few days. Drowsiness can be also due to:

- other medications, especially antidepressants, tranquil-lizers and antiemetics;
- metabolic disturbances, especially hypercalcemia, renal and hepatic failure;
- brain metastases;
- respiratory failure;
- end-stage disease.

If drowsiness develops in a patient who has been on opioids for some time, other causes of sedation or reasons for opioid toxicity such as decreased renal clearance should be looked for.

Prolonged drowsiness beyond 3 to 4 days or severe drowsiness with any dose may require some decrease in opioid dosage. If this fails to relieve sedation, then one should search for another correctable cause. In patients whose function is severely affected by opioid-related drowsiness, an amphetamine-like drug such as methylphenidate, given 5 to 10 mg 2 to 3 times a day, may have to be prescribed. Amphetamines can be associated with psychotomimetic problems and patients need to be monitored. CNS-stimulant drugs must not be used in patients with confusion, paranoia or delirium. Sometimes, switching from one opioid drug to another may alleviate drowsiness.

Confusion

Confusion can occur, especially in elderly patients. Their families and caregivers should be warned about the possibility of mild confusion in the first few days. Again, other factors causing confusion should be looked for and corrected as necessary. Small doses of major tranquilizers (e.g., haloperidol, 0.5 to 5 mg daily) may be helpful. Severe confusion related to opioids may require a significant decrease in opioid dose with a very gradual reintroduction of the drug or a switch to another strong opioid.

Psychotomimetic Effects

In some patients, dysphoria, hallucinations and nightmares might accompany the use of opioids. Generally these are minimal, but they can be very distressing to the patient and family. Reassurance is usually all that is necessary, although major and minor tranquilizers might prove to be beneficial in patients with severe or intolerable symptoms. Switching to another opioid drug may be required.

Respiratory Depression

Although much feared by many caregivers, respiratory depression is very seldom seen in patients taking opioids for the long term. Respiratory depression can occur when the opioid dose is much too high at the beginning, when increases are made too rapidly, or when the increments are too large for patients with chronic obstructive pulmonary disease or other major respiratory problems. It may also occur in patients with renal failure, in patients who are septic, and in patients receiving too-high or too-frequent parenteral doses of strong opioids. Very rarely, some patients have an idiosyncratic reaction to opioids that manifests as extreme sensitivity to the respiratory-depressant effect.

Use of an opioid antagonist such as naloxone should be avoided unless respiratory depression is very severe (for example, a respiratory rate less than 6 per minute). When naloxone must be used, it should be prescribed in smaller doses, such as 0.1 mg intravenously every 5 to 10 minutes, until the respiratory rate has increased to above 10 per minute. Vigorous use of higher doses of naloxone might cause reversal of analgesic effect, prolonged blockade of opiate receptors and severe pain that is difficult to control.

Myoclonus

Multifocal myoclonus is seen most often at higher doses of strong opioids, though in some patients it can be seen even at low doses. Usually, only an explanation to the patient is required. However, in severe cases these sudden muscular contractions can increase pain, especially bone pain. Also, the patient might find frequent muscle contractions disturbing. Frequent myoclonus is also a sign of opioid toxicity, which can be controlled by decreasing the dose or switching to a different opioid. Lorazepam, midazolam, clonazepam, baclofen, dantrolene and diazepam can be effective in decreasing myoclonus in usual doses, and they should be tried if the decreased dose of opioid exposes the patient to unacceptable levels of pain.

Urinary Retention

Urinary retention is uncommon and most often occurs in the elderly, especially men, because opioids increase bladder sphincter tone. Urinary retention might also be due to bladder outlet obstruction, fecal impaction, and drugs with anticholinergic effects such as antidepressants and antiemetics. Urinary retention due to opioids alone is usually incomplete and transient but, in some patients, a urinary catheter may be necessary.

Dry Mouth

Dry mouth is fairly frequent when strong opioids are used. The problem is complicated by dry mouth from other factors, such as dehydration, other medications (such as tricyclic antidepressants), oral candidiasis, post-chemotherapy mucositis and decreased salivary flow as a result of radiation. The best treatment comprises frequent intake of oral fluids and sugar-free candies, treatment of candidiasis and careful attention to oral hygiene. Alcohol-containing mouthwashes are best avoided because they can irritate and further dry the oral mucosa.

Miscellaneous Uncommon Side Effects

The following side effects are relatively uncommon, but are seen with all strong opioids:

- sweating;
- pruritus;
- postural hypotension;
- vertigo.

Patients with Infection or Sepsis

For some unexplained reason, patients who develop severe infections or sepsis can suddenly develop opioid toxicity. This is usually manifested by increased sedation, confusion, nausea and myoclonus. Such patients often require only a reduction or withholding of opioids until toxicity disappears. Occasionally patients will develop respiratory depression, and naloxone should be administered as previously discussed (p. 70).

10 Alternative Methods of Administering Opioids

The oral route is preferred for administering opioids because of the ease of administration in all settings, but physical and psychologic issues in some patients may preclude the use of oral medication.

Alternative routes of administration of opioids should be considered in the following circumstances.

- **Oral administration is not possible because patients cannot swallow.** Dysphagia may occur from obstructing pharyngeal or esophageal tumors, pharyngeal neuromuscular incoordination, extreme drowsiness or coma, and extreme weakness. Very confused or agitated patients may not be able to take oral medication well.

- **Intestinal obstruction occurs.** Most patients with complete unremitting gastrointestinal obstruction may not be able to take oral medications.

- **Patients are in the very terminal phase of their lives.** Factors such as severe weakness and decreased level of consciousness may make oral administration a problem during the last few days or hours of a patient's life. Parenteral administration is the major alternative.

- **Intractable adverse effects, especially nausea and vomiting, occur.** Some patients have intractable nausea despite maximum treatment with antiemetics, making oral opioid administration impractical; such patients can be transferred to parenteral opioid therapy.

- **Extremely severe pain requires urgent management.** Occasionally, patients experience a pain crisis requiring urgent and rapid management of pain. This type of suffering cannot wait for control by the generally slower oral route. When pain is finally controlled, the oral route may be tried again.

- **Psychologic issues are evident.** Some patients have an extreme aversion to oral opioids. Severe anxiety or some cognitive dysfunction may cause compliance problems that may be solved by alternative routes of administration.

- **There is poor compliance with analgesic medication.** Some routes of administration may be more effective for patients who have compliance problems.

Regular Parenteral Injections

Opioids should generally be administered subcutaneously, rarely intramuscularly. In patients who are at the end of life and may only require a few regular injections over a 12- to 24-hour period, opioids can be given every 3 to 4 hours by intermittent subcutaneous injections, in as concentrated a form as possible, using small gauge needles.

If injections are needed for a few days, consideration should be given to inserting a small-gauge butterfly needle subcutaneously, held in place with a clear occlusive dressing. Regular injections by this route can be given every 3 to 4 hours. This technique is much less expensive and less complex than using a continuous, subcutaneous-infusion pump; however, it may not be appropriate if very large doses of opioids and injected volumes such as 5 to 10 mL are required. Also, side effects such as nausea and sedation secondary to peak effects of bolus dosing may be more common with this method. The injection site may need to be changed every 3 to 10 days as necessary.

Continuous Subcutaneous Infusion

Continuous subcutaneous-infusion devices have been recently developed to provide an alternative method of administering opioids. Such devices may be syringe drivers, portable pumps with special medication cassettes or disposable constant-infusion hydraulic devices. These devices have proved to be extremely valuable, but their use should be discouraged in situations where the oral or other routes have not been given an adequate trial. Only about 5 percent of patients probably require infusion as the primary method of opioid administration. Most devices can be programmed to give a constant rate of infusion but allow for bolus breakthrough doses as well.

The pumps can be used for prolonged periods in institutions or at home. Service providers should be very familiar with the operation of infusion devices. Patient and family need careful education and 24-hour back-up if the pumps are to be managed successfully at home.

Consideration should be given to cost, especially in provinces where equipment, dispensing costs, etc. are not covered by health insurance.

Continuous Intravenous Infusion

Continuous intravenous infusion of morphine can also be a valuable technique, but usually can be managed only in a hospital because it requires considerable monitoring, specialized equipment and maintenance of intravenous sites. Its advantage over alternative methods, particularly continuous subcutaneous infusion, has never been demonstrated. Therefore, the use of continuous intravenous infusion is not generally indicated.

Epidural Opioids

Opioids can be administered through an epidural catheter to produce analgesia. Small doses of morphine can produce profound and long-lasting effects by this route, but the technique requires special equipment and experienced, trained personnel. The epidural route may have an infrequent role in certain localized, intractable pain syndromes. Its efficacy over other methods has never been conclusively demonstrated; therefore, it is not recommended as a primary method of opioid administration. Epidurals can be managed in home care situations if the family can be trained well to monitor pain and administer medications. Intermittent injections or constant infusions may be used. Preservative-free solutions are required. Catheters for chronic epidural administration of opioids should be tunneled under the skin to minimize the accidental removal of the catheter. Complications of epidural catheters include infection, blockage of the catheter, and respiratory depression from diffusion of opioid up towards the respiratory centre.

Rectal Suppositories

Immediate-release and controlled-release rectal suppositories of opioids can be effective when the oral route is not possible. Patients and family members should be educated about the appropriate use of rectal suppositories and their concerns about this route of administration should be addressed. Rectal suppositories can provide emergency support when constant infusion devices pose technical problems. Recently, a controlled-release morphine suppository has been made available (see Table 8 on p. 45 for available strengths). The twice-daily dosing frequency may be more acceptable to patients than the q4h immediate-release form. The conversion ratio of controlled-release morphine tablets to controlled-release morphine suppositories is usually 1:1.[1]

Sublingual Opioids

Efficacy of sublingual administration of morphine is neither well documented nor proved. Morphine is poorly absorbed across oral membranes. Hydromorphone may be better absorbed. High-concentration liquid morphine preparations (20 to 50 mg/mL) and hydromorphone liquid can be effective; however, this may be a result of swallowing morphine rather than sublingual or transmucosal absorption. The use of sublingual or buccal morphine for a few doses in drowsy or comatose patients may be appropriate at the very end of life. Sublingual morphine is carefully delivered, drop by drop. Immediate-release tablets can be dissolved in a little water and administered gradually by dropper sublingually or buccally. Sublingual fentanyl is a possible option that is under study.

Buprenorphine, a very potent agonist-antagonist opioid, is well absorbed as a sublingual preparation, but it is available only in the United Kingdom. It probably offers no advantages and, as an agonist-antagonist, has considerable disadvantages.

Transdermal Fentanyl

Transdermal fentanyl is a unique delivery system for opioids and offers an alternative, non-invasive method of controlling pain for selected patients. This technique of opioid administration has value in patients who:

- cannot take oral medication because of difficulties swallowing;
- cannot tolerate oral opioids because of intractable side effects.

Problems in dose equivalence and slow achievement of a steady state preclude the use of transdermal fentanyl in patients who have severe, unstable pain that needs rapid control, or in patients who have a life expectancy of less than a few hours or days.

After the patch is applied, a plateau level of the drug is seen after 12 to 24 hours. There is also a skin depot of medication so that removing the patch results in very gradual elimination of the drug; it can take close to 24 hours to reach 50 percent of the plateau level.[2] This may lead to prolonged adverse effects, even after the patch is removed. Each patch is usually effective for 72 hours, but infrequently the patch may need to be changed as often as every 48 hours. It is recommended that total dosage be changed only every 72 hours. Breakthrough pain in the 72-hour interval must be handled using an immediate-release opioid such as morphine or hydromorphone. The spectrum of adverse effects is the same as for other strong opioids. The fentanyl patch has a recommended ceiling dose of 300 µg/hr, but higher doses may sometimes be used.

Patch care and placement is important. The patch needs to be applied to hairless, clean and dry skin. Firm pressure must be applied after application, for about a minute. Some patients experience difficulty with adhesion of the patch to the skin. In patients who have major problems of adhesion, another method of opioid administration should be sought.

Table 17: Conversion of Oral Morphine to Transdermal Fentanyl*

ORAL MORPHINE (mg/day)	FENTANYL (μg/hr)	ORAL MORPHINE (mg/day)	FENTANYL (μg/hr)
30 to 90	25	391 to 450	175
91 to 150	50	451 to 510	200
151 to 210	75	511 to 570	225
211 to 270	100	571 to 630	250
271 to 330	125	631 to 690	275
331 to 390	150	691 to 750	300

Modified after Donner and Zenz[3]

* approximately 50 percent of patients will require further dose increases after conversion to transdermal fentanyl

References

1. Bruera E, Fainsinger R, Spachynski K et al. Clinical efficacy and safety of a novel controlled-release morphine suppository and subcutaneous morphine in cancer pain: A randomized evaluation. *J Clin Oncol* 1995; 13:1520-7.

2. Mosser KH. Transdermal fentanyl in cancer pain. *Am Fam Phys* 1992; 45: 2289-94.

3. Donner B, Zenz M. Transdermal fentanyl: a new step on the therapeutic ladder. *Anti-Cancer Drugs* 1995; 6:39-43.

11 *Adjuvant Therapy*

Adjuvants (adjuncts) to control cancer pain must be considered at all stages of the patient's cancer. There may be very specific treatments that are effective and have minimal adverse effects. Some adjuvants will be effective in relaxing the patient and enhancing pain control. Other pain treatments may reduce the medication load for patients and reduce the risk of adverse drug reactions.

Adjuvant Pharmacotherapy

Bone pain. Always consider the use of NSAIDs when bone metastases cause pain. See pp. 32-33.

Neuropathic pain. Pain from nerve compression or destruction can be very difficult to control. It may be only partially responsive to morphine and other opioids. Nevertheless, a trial of opioids is necessary because the pain has a number of components of which neuropathic pain is but one. When a patient with neuropathic, opioid-resistant pain develops increasing drowsiness or side effects as the opioid dose is increased, the limit of usefulness of opioid for that pain has probably been reached. Other medications can then be very useful in controlling neuropathic pain.

- **Glucocorticosteroids.** Prednisone (20 to 60 mg daily reducing to 10 mg) according to response, and particularly dexamethasone (16 mg reducing to 4 mg daily), can be helpful for nerve compression pain. Glucocorticosteroids may work by reducing perineural edema.

- **Antidepressants.** Tricyclic antidepressants, such as imipramine, amitriptyline and others, may be very useful in managing dysesthetic pain caused by nerve destruction. Serotonin-specific re-uptake inhibitors (SSRIs), a newer class of antidepressants, generally have not been shown to have much analgesic activity. Only paroxetine has shown some early promise of analgesic efficacy.

There is no definite optimum dose, although a trial of the tricyclic agents should begin with a small dose (25 mg) at bedtime and work upwards, according to response and side effects, to a dose of 100 to 150 mg (Table 18), after which little response can be expected. Desipramine and imipramine are usually less sedating than amitriptyline. Relief may be expected within 1 to 2 weeks of maximum dosage. The adverse effects of these tricyclic antidepressants, specifically sedation, dry mouth and urinary retention (anticholinergic effects), may limit their dosage and their usefulness, especially in elderly patients.

Table 18: Antidepressants for Neuropathic Pain

DRUGS	DOSAGE	COMMENTS
Cyclic Drugs		
Amitriptyline Imipramine Maprotiline Desipramine Nortriptyline	Begin with 25 mg and increase gradually to 150 mg h.s.	Adverse effects often limit use
SSRIs		
Paroxetine	20 to 40 mg h.s.	Some sedation may occur

- **Anticonvulsant medication.** Several anticonvulsant medications can be helpful in managing the pain of nerve destruction. A full response may take up to 2 to 3 weeks, but some change in the pain may be seen after 4 to 5 days. The most useful agents seem to be valproic acid and carbamazepine (Table 19).

Table 19: Anticonvulsants for Neuropathic Pain

DRUGS	DOSAGE	ADVERSE EFFECTS	COMMENTS
Valproic acid	250 to 500 mg h.s. increasing to 1000 to 1500 mg h.s.	Sedation Rarely, thrombo-cytopenia	Blood levels should be monitored
Carbamazepine	100 to 200 mg b.i.d. increasing slowly to a maximum of 400 mg t.i.d.	Drowsiness Nausea Interaction with antidepressants may increase effects of both	Blood levels should be monitored
Phenytoin	Up to 600 mg once daily		Little data on use Blood levels should be monitored
Gabapentin	300 to 900 mg starting at 300 mg once daily and increasing to 300 mg t.i.d.	Sedation	New agent
Clonazepam	0.5 mg h.s. increasing to 2 to 3 mg daily	Drowsiness common and limiting	May be useful

- **Membrane-stabilizing agents.** Drugs such as flecainide and mexiletine (Table 20, p. 82) are local anesthetic congeners used mainly in cardiac dysrhythmias. Recent research has shown that these agents may be useful in neuropathic pain, but they should be used carefully in patients with cardiac disease. An ECG is warranted before beginning treatment to check for conduction disturbances. The use of membrane stabilizers should be reserved for neuropathic pain that has resisted other efforts at control. A palliative care or pain consultant should be consulted before using these drugs.

Table 20: Membrane-Stabilizing Drugs for Neuropathic Pain

DRUGS	DOSAGE	ADVERSE EFFECTS	COMMENTS
Mexiletine	Start with 50 to 100 mg b.i.d. and increase gradually to 600 mg daily	Nausea CNS effects, e.g., confusion, ataxia, tremors	Cannot be used with tricyclic antidepressants
Flecainide	Start with 50 mg b.i.d. and increase every 5 to 7 days to a maximum of 150 mg b.i.d.	CNS effects fairly common, e.g., confusion, drowsiness, agitation; rarely, seizures	Cannot be used with tricyclic antidepressants

- **Bisphosphonates.** Bisphosphonates are inorganic pyrophosphate analogues that inhibit osteoclast-mediated bone resorption. These agents have been used extensively in the treatment of hypercalcemia associated with malignancies. They also may have some effect on bone pain in normocalcemic patients with bone metastases. Drugs such as clodronate, pamidronate or etidronate may be useful in some patients (especially those with widespread breast, prostate or lung cancer) with bone pain refractory to opioids, radiation or NSAIDs. Side effects are generally minimal although there is the risk of significant hypocalcemia.

  In general, it is recommended that bisphosphonate therapy be supervised by a palliative care or cancer pain expert.

- **Tranquilizers.** Major or minor tranquilizers may be extremely useful when patients with advanced cancer display symptoms of anxiety. However, the use of tranquilizers is no substitute for assessing a patient and family for the source of anxiety and providing appropriate counselling along with the drugs. In an anxious patient with pain, tranquilizers are not an adequate substitute for analgesics. Pain will rarely if ever be controlled by tranquilizers alone. For the most part, benzodiazepines should be used (Table 21). Benzodiazepines may be useful in reducing muscle spasm that may contribute to pain. Major tranquilizers should be used for anxiety only if benzodiazepines are not effective, or if the patient is severely agitated.

Table 21: Useful Tranquilizers

Drugs	Dosage	Comments
Benzodiazepines		
Lorazepam	0.5 to 2 mg q4h to q8h p.o. 1 to 2 mg i.v. if urgent situation	Can accumulate because of relatively long half-life
Oxazepam	15 to 30 mg t.i.d.	Long half-life may cause accumulation and drowsiness
Diazepam	5 to 10 mg p.o. b.i.d. to t.i.d.	Longest-acting and may cause prolonged drowsiness
Midazolam	5 to 30 mg per day i.v. or s.c.	Can be used in s.c. infusions; short-acting; narrow range of safety
Triazolam	0.125 mg to 0. 5 mg h.s.	Hypnotic; may cause amnesia especially in elderly
Alprazolam	0.25 mg to 0. 5 mg b.i.d. to t.i.d.	Short-acting; least sedating
Major Tranquilizers		
Haloperidol	0.5 to 5.0 mg b.i.d. or t.i.d. p.o. or s.c.	Extrapyramidal side effects common at higher dosages and with prolonged use
Chlorpromazine	25 to 50 mg q4 to 6h p.o. or i.m.	May cause drowsiness; extrapyramidal effects common
Loxapine	5 to 10 mg p.o. or i.m. q4 to 6h	Needs careful titration but probably most effective for severe agitation or in organic psychosis

■ **Nitrous oxide inhalation.** Patients who have very severe pain on movement, for example, from major pathologic fractures or changing dressing in painful wounds, may respond to analgesic inhalations of nitrous oxide using an inhaling device (such as a nitrous oxide inhaler) when they need to be moved in bed.

Radiotherapy

Palliative radiotherapy is an important adjunct in the treatment of cancer pain. For bone pain, it should be considered the initial treatment of choice unless the patient's disease is very far advanced, if transportation to a radiotherapy centre would be very difficult, or if the patient has already had maximum radiation to the area involved. Radiotherapy may also help to relieve pain from spinal cord compression, pain secondary to brain metastases or to tumor pressing on nerves. It usually will not be effective in nerve-destruction pain.

In metastatic cancer to bone, a recent adjuvant and palliative treatment involves the use of Strontium-89. This radioactive isotope seems to bind preferentially to osteoblastic metastatic sites. It has been found to be most useful in prostatic cancer and in breast cancer.

Cancer Chemotherapy

If the patient's cancer responds to chemotherapy, pain may be improved considerably. For example, a patient with liver pain may gain considerable relief as a result of the reduction in size of the tumors and decreased stretch on the liver capsule, which is the usual source of pain. Breast cancer metastases may respond dramatically to hormonal therapies and pain may disappear. Unfortunately, in many cancer trials the issue of pain control has not been addressed directly and there are often too many co-interventions, such as opioid use, and supportive interventions that complicate the estimation of causal relationships between chemotherapy and pain control. The patient's pain should always be treated aggressively and should not be delayed until the results of chemotherapy are known.

Neurosurgical Procedures

Occasionally, patients may benefit by neuroablative procedures such as cordotomy to interrupt pain pathways in the spinal cord. These procedures are beneficial mainly to those with well-localized unilateral upper and lower limb pain or unilateral pelvic pain. Patients may develop disabling secondary neuropathic pain several weeks or months after these procedures or, rarely, motor weakness or bladder and bowel sphincter problems.

Nerve Blocks

Nerve blocks may be helpful in a small number of patients when other methods have failed an adequate trial. However, nerve blocks require specialized personnel and equipment. Blocks may be more permanent neurolytic blocks or temporary blocks with local anesthetic agents.

Celiac plexus neurolytic blocks can be helpful with pancreatic, gastric or liver cancers. Caudal blocks in the sacral canal may alleviate sciatic, perineal or pelvic pain.

In severe abdominal, pelvic or lower-limb pain that has not responded to all other measures, consideration should be given to an epidural block using a local anesthetic such as bupivacaine. This, of course, may cause motor weakness and numbness below the level of the block, but in the patient exhausted by severe pain epidural block may provide the only relief while other measures are being considered.

Physiotherapy and Occupational Therapy

The physiotherapist and occupational therapists can provide special care to patients to assist them in conserving energy, minimizing incident pain, relieving muscle spasm, preserving function and using special aids appropriately. These therapists are invaluable in making functional assessments of patients so that home care needs can be assessed. Even patients with advanced cancer can benefit from active rehabilitation.

Other Complementary Therapies

There are a variety of other non-drug therapies for pain. Some of them are considered "alternative" or complementary therapies because scientific evidence about their effectiveness is often lacking. Dismissing such treatments because there is no good scientific proof of their efficacy is not justified; much of the conventional medical care we now use and find effective has never been tested by rigorous scientific trials. These techniques may be helpful adjuncts to pain control.

We do know that some techniques—acupuncture and transcutaneous nerve stimulation—produce physiologic changes such as the release of endogenous opioids, but there are many parts to the pain puzzle that still need to be solved before we can say for certain how those techniques produce an effect.

Many cancer patients will seek out unconventional or non-traditional forms of treatment. The clinician must not only be able to listen to the patient's concerns and wishes, without being too judgmental, but also be careful to advise patients about potentially harmful therapy. Most of the common, alternative treatments for cancer pain are not quackery and their practitioners do not advise patients to eschew more traditional forms of treatment. Most of the techniques listed below are given in conjunction with more standard forms of therapy. However, patients need to be warned about the charlatan who advertises or advises that cancer can be cured with a particular unorthodox technique (usually at high cost) or who advises the cessation of proven therapies.

Physical Approaches

- **Acupuncture** does have effect in a variety of painful conditions. Its use in cancer pain has never been thoroughly studied. Acupuncture is probably best given by a practitioner who has considerable experience in modern techniques of this therapy. Anecdotal evidence suggests that acupuncture is of little use in neuropathic pain.

- **Hypnosis** may help a patient cope with pain, but it will rarely control all aspects of severe pain. It may be useful as an adjunct in the hands of a skilled practitioner.

- **Transcutaneous electrical nerve stimulation (TENS)** may be helpful in some cases of regional pain, but many patients develop rapid resistance to it. Use of newer techniques such as the Codetron TENS apparatus may prove to be more beneficial but there is a need for good research in this area.

- **Chiropractic and manipulation** are not recommended in the presence of bone metastases.

- **Massage therapy.** Here as well, there is a need for further research.

Psychologic Approaches

- **Relaxation techniques** are often helpful adjuncts in the treatment of pain to reduce associated anxiety and tension, as are imagery, biofeedback, and therapeutic touch. However, effects have not as yet been clearly documented in research data.

Other Approaches

Such approaches include herbal therapy, aromatherapy, and homeopathy. Uses in cancer pain have not been thoroughly studied, however.

12 Special Problems in Pain Control

Overwhelming Pain

Occasionally, patients experience rapidly increasing pain or have severe pain that they or their physician have neglected. Physicians must recognize that this pain is an emergency and requires immediate relief. A parenteral opioid should be tried first, with rapid increase in the dose until the pain is better controlled. As the dose of opioid gets higher, sedation may provide welcome relief, but other sedatives may also be needed. Obviously, the patient must be monitored carefully and often. Unfortunately, the pain in these situations is often resistant to opioids.

Every effort must be made to determine the cause of the overwhelming pain as quickly as possible. Rapidly increasing back pain, with or without neurologic signs, may be a clue to compression of the spinal cord. Immediate investigation using CT myelogram or MRI, followed by radiation and possibly surgery, may be required to prevent neurologic problems such as paraplegia. Sudden, excruciating limb pain may signal a major unstable fracture (e.g., fractured long bone). Patients should be referred to an orthopedic consultant to determine if stabilization and surgical repair are possible.

When pain does become overwhelming, physicians should consult with the patient and family to determine the best course. Consultation with palliative-care and pain-control specialists is also mandatory. Nitrous oxide inhalation or intense sedation should be considered.

Intractable Pain

Severe unrelenting and unresponsive pain, in spite of intensive efforts at control, is serious but fortunately rare. All the factors constituting total pain (pp. 11-12) must be re-examined, and a team approach involving experts in pain control is essential. If the patient is in the very last stages of the illness, intense sedation may be the only answer, but this should be administered only after consultation with the patient, family and all members of the treatment team.

Bowel Obstruction

Bowel obstruction commonly complicates all types of intra-abdominal malignancies, and surgery is frequently impossible because of the diffuseness of the disease and the patient's condition. However, the patient's pain and nausea can be managed at home or in institutions without uncomfortable nasogastric suction and intravenous fluids. A constant subcutaneous infusion of morphine plus scopolamine butylbromide (50 to 100 mg daily) and haloperidol (5 to 15 mg daily) may abolish or reduce nausea to tolerable levels. Another approach involves opioids to control pain, along with oral loperamide, 2 to 8 mg every 4 to 6 hours. Octreotide 100 to 500 µg daily will also reduce gastrointestinal secretions in those patients with intractable obstruction. Patients who are being cared for at home and who wish to receive supplementary fluids can be given fluids via hypodermoclysis instead of the more problematic intravenous route.

Patients should be assessed daily because bowel obstruction is often intermittent. However, the obstruction may be totally irreversible, and physicians must maintain good communication with the patient and family to prepare them for the patient's progressive decline and ultimate demise.

In bowel-obstructed patients, oral administration of immediate-release opioids may be possible especially if patients are vomiting infrequently. Controlled-action opioids are not recommended. If the oral route is not possible, alternative routes of administration should be used (see Chapter 10, p. 73).

Compliance Problems

Although one would assume that patients with chronic cancer pain are careful to take their pain medication faithfully, no studies confirm this. Indeed, at times patients do not comply with the prescribed therapy, possibly because they have emotional, cognitive or family problems, or because they have extreme fear or aversion to medication. A few may not comply deliberately to gain more attention and sympathy from caregivers and family. Some compliance problems may relate to a patient's memory problems or other cognitive dysfunction. Sometimes patients do not follow a prescribed regimen but adapt it to suit their need to be in control.

Compliance problems must always be considered if a patient's pain is not responding to medication or the pain reappears suddenly for no apparent reason.

Extremely rarely, a patient may reject all forms of pain treatment. Service providers must always remember that their own philosophy or perception of quality of life may be different from the patient's, and they must be prepared to listen carefully to the patient's point of view, to accept it, and to continue providing empathetic care.

The Conspiracy of Silence

Occasionally, physicians and other caregivers are involved in treating patients who truly are not aware of their advanced cancer. This type of situation usually arises when a family attempts to "protect" the patient, thinking that the truth may, in some way, be harmful. However, the patient may once have stated that, if cancer were ever found, he or she did not want to be told. Also, some cultural groups do not routinely disclose a diagnosis of cancer. Very often the patient does know most of the truth and is trying to protect the family. A family meeting can quickly clarify the issues.

Management of pain under such circumstances can be very difficult. Patients may reject strong opioids because they believe their illness is benign and they fear addiction. They may question why they have pain and, if they ask for an explanation, the physicians or caregivers are caught in an ethical dilemma—the only way to maintain the conspiracy of silence is by lying to the patient.

A careful team approach to exploring with the family its reasons and fears about telling the patient the truth may resolve the situation and allow the team to plan care that meets the family's and the patient's needs.

When Fluid Intake Decreases

Maintenance of fluid intake will often become a problem in patients who are becoming very debilitated. They may be simply too weak to drink very much. Nasogastric feeding may help, but it is rarely necessary, and the nasogastric tube is an additional source of discomfort and bother to both patients and family. The use of intravenous fluids needs to be discussed carefully with everyone involved, but usually the patients can be managed well only in an institution. For end-stage patients, hypodermoclysis, administration of crystalloid fluids subcutaneously, with or without hyaluronidase, can be managed at home. In some patients with a relatively long prognosis and with decreased intake due to pharyngeal, esophageal or gastric obstruction, insertion of a feeding tube through the abdominal wall under imaging guidance will provide an alternate route for food and fluids.

Service providers should discuss with patients and their family the rationale for no longer needing to maintain fluid intake in the face of imminent death. The discomfort associated with dehydration is probably more an emotional problem for onlookers than a physical or emotional one for patients. They may tolerate minimal fluids as long as they are given aggressive mouth care for comfort. Other methods of administration of analgesics will need to be considered at this time (see Chapter 10, p. 73).

Metabolic Problems in Advanced Cancer

The course of advanced cancer may be complicated by metabolic problems such as renal failure, hepatic failure, hypercalcemia and inappropriate secretion of antidiuretic and other hormones. Treatment of these conditions in patients with very advanced disease should be decided by the patients, family and caregivers. The option of no treatment should be discussed openly and with the understanding that physical discomfort can be kept at a minimum in most situations.

AIDS/HIV Disease and Pain

Acquired immune deficiency syndrome (AIDS) and conditions caused by the human immunodeficiency virus (HIV) may be accompanied by pain that is often severe.[1,2] Some results of a recent study from France[3] on the prevalence of pain with AIDS/HIV disease are outlined in Table 22. Many patients with AIDS/HIV infection have severe pain.

Table 22: Prevalence of Pain in AIDS/HIV Disease Patients

Pain as Symptom*	
Mechanism	*Prevalence (%)*
Neuropathic	21
Digestive	17
Muscular	15
Infectious	14
Bone and joint	10
Iatrogenic	4
Psychogenic	3
Cancer/tumor	1
Unknown	5

*experienced by 52% of patients

Most issues in pain management in AIDS/HIV disease are the same as in managing pain from cancer, but there are a few issues that need highlighting.

- The oral route of administration is preferred in order to minimize the exposure of service providers and other caregivers to the risk of needle-stick injury and other exposure to contaminated blood.

- Controlled-release opioids can be useful but should not be used in patients with diarrhea (for example, from cryptosporidium).[4]

- Any episode of serious acute infection may lead to opioid toxicity. Patients in such acute infectious processes may need to be monitored very carefully.

- Patients early on in the course of their AIDS/HIV disease can be maintained on long-term potent opioids. The severity of pain should guide treatment, not the duration of treatment nor the concerns physicians have about long-term use.

- In the subpopulation of substance abusers with AIDS/HIV disease, the treatment of pain may be more difficult. The help of specialists such as palliative care consultants and addiction consultants can be helpful. The approach should be one that emphasizes harm reduction to lessen the amount of risk to everyone from drug-seeking behaviors, parenteral use of drugs, and other social and behavioral aspects of substance abuse[5].

- In hemophiliacs who have contracted AIDS/HIV disease from contaminated blood products, acute joint pain from intra-articular bleeding will require potent opioids for control.

- Adverse effects from opioids in those who have AIDS/HIV disease are similar to such adverse effects in other patients. However, patients with cognitive dysfunction may be more sensitive to the psychotomimetic effects of opioids.

- Cognitive dysfunction is common in patients with AIDS/HIV disease. Drug regimens should extensively utilize oral controlled-release opioid preparations on a 12-hourly basis, or other alternative routes in order to simplify drug administration and to minimize risk from poor compliance.

References

1.   Breitbart W, McDonald MV, Rosenfeld B et al. Pain in ambulatory AIDS patients. I: Pain characteristics and medical correlates. *Pain* 1996; 68:315-21.

2.   Rosenfeld B, Breitbart W, McDonald MV et al. Pain in ambulatory AIDS patients. II: Impact of pain on psychological functioning and quality of life. *Pain* 1996; 68:323-328.

3.   Larue F, Brasseur L, Musseault et al. Pain and symptoms during HIV disease. A French national study. *J Palliative Care* 1994; 10:95.

4.   Dixon P, Higginson I. AIDS and cancer pain treated with slow-release morphine. *Postgrad Med J* 1991; 67:S92-S94.

5.   Ferris FD, Flannery JS, McNeal HB, Morisette MR, Cameron R, Bally GA (eds). *A Comprehensive Guide for the Care of Persons with HIV Disease. Module 4: Palliative Care.* Mount Sinai Hospital and Casey House Hospice, Toronto, 1995: 110-13.

13 Cancer Pain in Children

The prevalence of cancer in children is fortunately quite low. However, children of all ages are probably as likely as adults to suffer from pain when they have cancer. Also, the procedures that children have to undergo during the investigation and treatment of their illness often are themselves quite painful and frightening and, therefore, heighten their total pain. Pain in children must be treated as vigorously as pain in adults.

Undertreatment of Pain in Children

Inadequate treatment of pain in children has been identified as a problem in all aspects of pediatric care.[1] The reasons for this are complex but include the following:

- Myths about the child's ability to feel and remember pain:
  - newborns and infants do not feel pain because their nervous systems are not mature;
  - infants do not remember pain, therefore analgesia is not needed because they will forget the pain and it will have no lasting effects;
  - children cry out of fear, not pain;
  - children need to learn to tolerate a little pain;
  - children can become addicted to opioids and therefore it is best not to expose them to potent opioids.
- Problems in pain assessment in children:
  - preverbal children;
  - differentiating anxiety or fear and pain;
  - poor knowledge by service providers about the assessment of pain in children.

- Failure to consider all components of "total pain":
  - other symptoms;
  - emotional distress;
  - cultural issues;
  - unsupportive parents and other family issues;
  - unsupportive service-provider environment;
  - frequent or chronic uncontrolled pain leading to "learned helplessness".

Cancer Pain Syndromes in Children

Cancer pain syndromes in children are similar to those in adults. A careful broad-based assessment that seeks out all problems that could lead to pain will clarify the types of pain and allow for effective management.

Pain Assessment in Children

The basic principles of pain assessment outlined in Chapter 3 (p. 19) are for the most part a reasonable guideline to assessing pain in children, with some important additions.

- The child's report of pain should always be believed. Pain should be expected when there are disease manifestations that should ordinarily lead to pain, e.g., bone metastases, massive splenomegaly or procedures that are known to cause pain. Denials of pain in such circumstances need careful investigation.

- The environment surrounding the child (family, community, school, hospital, clinic) should be conducive to assessing and monitoring pain. This requires a commitment in all those locations to the assessment and effective management of a child's pain. Service providers need to be educated about children's pain.

- In children under 3 years of age, behavioral indicators of pain are of prime importance. Table 23 provides a checklist for assessing degree of pain.

Table 23: Checklist for Behavioral Indicators in Children

BEHAVIOR	NOT PRESENT	PRESENT
Crying	☐	☐
Fussing, irritability	☐	☐
Withdrawal from social interaction	☐	☐
Sleep disturbance	☐	☐
Facial grimacing	☐	☐
Guarding	☐	☐
Not easily consoled	☐	☐
Reduction in play	☐	☐
Reduction in attention span	☐	☐

Adapted from McGrath PJ, Beyer J, Cleeland C et al. Report of the subcommittee on assessment and methodological issues in the management of pain in childhood cancer. *Pediatrics* 1990: 86; 814-7. Copyright 1990. With permission.

As in adults, an observed behavior may have many underlying factors including the disease or treatment (e.g., reduction in eating). However, one must have a high index of suspicion of pain when such behaviors are observed.

In neonates, the observation of facial activity and type of cry combined with assessment of body movements does provide a reliable assessment tool in the hands of trained and experienced observers.[2]

■ Physiologic signs of pain such as heart rate, blood pressure, sweaty palms and respiratory rate are often affected by many other circumstances of the illness and its treatment, and are thus of secondary importance in assessing pain in children 3 to 6 years of age.

■ In children 3 to 6 years of age, special scales utilizing pictures such as the "Faces Pain Scale"[3] can be used to help understand the severity of the child's pain (Figure 6, p. 98).

- In children over 6 years of age, the self-reports of the child's pain are the best guide to the assessment of pain. An adequate pain history is essential. The language used with the child must of course be appropriate to his or her age, social environment and education. Visual analog scales similar to those in adults may be used effectively.

- Parents and other caregivers should be involved closely in the assessment and monitoring of pain. They need to be properly educated to do this. Pain diaries can be helpful.

- Assessment of adverse effects of medications by children is somewhat limited. The effect on quality of life, especially in younger children, is difficult to appraise.

Figure 6: The "Faces Pain Scale"

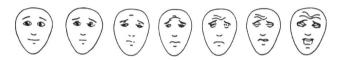

Numbers 0 to 6, left to right.

From Bieri D, Reeve RA, Champion GO et al. The Faces Pain Scale for the self-assessment of the severity of pain experienced by children: development, initial validation, and preliminary investigation for ratio scale properties. *Pain* 1990; 41:139-50. With kind permission from Elsevier Science-NL, Sara Burgerhartstraat 25, 1055 KV Amsterdam, the Netherlands.

Pain Management in Children

Pain in children should be managed as aggressively as pain in adults. The basic principles as outlined in Chapter 4 (p. 26) mostly apply to the effective management of children's pain. Pain management relies on effective treatment of the cancer, management of painful procedures, appropriate use of analgesics and pertinent use of adjuvant therapy. The pain management plan for each child should be very individualized.

Special issues in children include the following:

■ The non-opioid of choice is probably acetaminophen. ASA and other NSAIDs are less favored because of bleeding problems, especially since many children have abnormal blood counts due to hematologic malignancies or aggressive chemotherapy. NSAIDs are rarely used in general pediatric care.

■ The analgesic ladder does apply but again severe pain must be treated early with potent analgesics.

■ Opioid analgesics should be given regularly and, in most cases, orally. Breakthrough doses are appropriate. Adverse effects should be treated aggressively. Oral liquid preparations may be most suitable for children.

■ Most adjuvant drugs have not been studied extensively in pediatric populations. Drugs of choice for neuropathic pain have generally been antidepressants, particularly imipramine, rather than anticonvulsants; there are, however, few studies.

■ Pain can be managed by family physicians and general pediatricians, but ongoing consultation with a pediatric anesthetist or oncologist with knowledge and experience in pediatric pain management is often necessary.

Table 24 (p. 100) reviews recommended pediatric dosages of analgesic and adjuvant drugs in the management of cancer pain.

Table 24: Recommended Pediatric Dosages of Analgesic and Adjuvant Drugs

MEDICATION	DOSE, ROUTE, FREQUENCY	COMMENTS
Non-Opioids		
Acetaminophen	10 to 15 mg/kg p.o. q4h	Ceiling dose; liver toxicity
NSAIDs		
ASA	10 to 15 mg/kg p.o. q4h	Can increase dose if severe inflammation
Choline magnesium salicylate	25 mg/kg p.o. q6 to 8h	
Naproxen	5 mg/kg q8 to 12h	
Ibuprofen	4 to 10 mg/kg p.o. q6 to 8h	
Opioids*†		
Codeine	0.5 to 1.0 mg/kg p.o. q4h	For mild to moderate pain only
Morphine (immediate-release)	0.2 to 0.4 mg/kg p.o. q4h 0.1 to 0.2 mg/kg s.c. q4h 0.5 to 0.6 mg s.c./hr infusion	
Hydromorphone	1/4 to 1/6 of morphine dose	Not much data in children
Fentanyl	Intravenous use for procedures	No reliable data on transdermal route in children
Methadone		Not recommended unless physician is expert in its use

Table 24: (cont'd)

MEDICATION	DOSE, ROUTE, FREQUENCY	COMMENTS
Other Drugs		
Imipramine	0.2 mg/kg h.s. and gradually increase weekly to 1 to 3 mg/kg h.s.	Most studied of the tricyclics
Carbamazepine	6 to 12 yr: begin with 100 mg and increase gradually	Blood levels must be monitored; experience in children less than 6 yr not documented; chewtabs available
Prochlorperazine	0.13 mg/kg i.m. 9 to 14 kg: 2.5 to 7 mg/day p.o./p.r. 14 to 18 kg: 5 to 10 mg/day p.o./p.r. 18 to 39 kg: 7.5 to 15 mg/day p.o./p.r.	Dystonic reactions and sedation
Haloperidol	Less than 6 yr.: 0.25 to 1.0 mg/day p.o./s.c.	Safety in children not established
Dimenhydrinate	2 to 6 yr.: 15 to 25 mg q6 to 8h p.o./p.r. 6 to 12 yr.: 25 to 50 mg q6 to 8h p.o./p.r.	Drowsiness a problem

* NB starting doses
† Opioids not recommended: meperidine, any agonist-antagonist (e.g., pentazocine)

Adapted from Berde C, Ablin A, Glazer J et al. Report of the Subcommittee on disease-related pain in childhood cancer. *Pediatrics* 1990; 86:818-25. Copyright 1990. With permission.

Summary

Children with cancer and pain require careful and aggressive management of their pain. For further information about the treatment of pediatric pain and other symptoms one may refer to literature on the topic.[4]

References

1.   Schecter NL. The undertreatment of pain in children: an overview. *Ped Clin N Am.* 1989; 36:781-94.

2.   Grunau VE, Johnston CC, Craig KD. Neonatal facial and cry responses to invasive and non-invasive procedures. *Pain* 1990; 42:295-305.

3.   Bieri D, Reeve RA, Champion GD et al. The Faces of Pain Scale for the self-assessment of the severity of pain experienced by children: development, initial validation, and preliminary investigation for ratio scale properties. *Pain* 1990; 41:139-50.

4.   Report of the Consensus Conference on the management of pain in childhood cancer. *Pediatrics* 1990; 86:S811-S34.

14 Chronic Non-Malignant Pain

The problem of cancer pain is relatively small compared with the much larger problem of chronic non-malignant pain. This chapter provides a brief guide to issues and procedures in managing patients with chronic non-malignant pain, which can be as severe as cancer pain.

The chronic pain of many illnesses causes large losses of human productivity[1,2] and lifelong suffering that seems never ending for those who are affected. The undertreatment of both acute and chronic pain has been well documented in scientific literature.[3] The use of strong opioids in treating such pain has been problematic for many physicians because of their extreme fear of addiction and other fears about the long-term effects of such strong drugs. Yet opioids can be used very successfully in selected patients with non-malignant pain.[4-7]

The assessment of pain and the principles of management and opioid therapy outlined in this manual can, with some modifications, be applied to the management of non-malignant pain. Important steps include the following.

■ **Doing an adequate pain assessment.** The patient's own description of pain, especially pain quality, will help in classifying pain. Many chronic pains seen are neuropathic in origin. A detailed medication history is important. Effect on activities of daily living will measure in part the suffering of such patients. A thorough psychosocial inquiry is absolutely essential. Careful documentation is also crucial.

■ **Performing a systematic examination** looking specifically for findings consistent with the pain complaint.

■ **Investigating wisely.** For instance, the inadequacy of spinal x-rays in determining the source of back pain has been well documented.

- **Restoring patient control, self-esteem and autonomy.** This will involve education of patient and family about the cause and management of pain, providing supportive counselling for patient and family, being an advocate for the patient as appropriate and avoiding becoming part of the problem. This latter issue can occur when physicians and other service providers become punitive or unhelpful by their attitudes and biases.

- **Treating the pain wisely.** Pain management involves the effective around-the-clock use of analgesics and all other appropriate modalities for pain management.

- **Close monitoring of patients** is essential.

- **A coordinated multidisciplinary approach** is preferred.

- Help should be sought from multidisciplinary pain clinics for problematic pain **early on** in the course of chronic pain.

Recently, the Alberta College of Physicians and Surgeons published practical guidelines for the management of chronic pain and the use of opioids in these patients.[8] The recommendations, with some modification, can be summarized as follows.

- An accurate diagnosis of pain should be established.

- A history of recent or remote substance abuse is a relatively strong contraindication.

- An adequate trial of non-opioid analgesics and other modalities should have been carried out without success.

- Only one physician should prescribe opioids.

- The World Health Organization analgesic ladder should guide the prescriber (see Figure 4, p. 28).

- Treatment of pain with opioids should be done as a well-monitored therapeutic clinical trial. The dose of opioid should be titrated upwards until maximum pain control is achieved, adverse effects are intolerable or signs of abuse are noted.

- A contract should be documented with the patient to delineate issues such as how much medication will be prescribed at a time, how often medications will be renewed, the process for dose escalation, the prohibition of any unauthorized dose escalation and the clear consequences of any breach of trust.

- The physician needs to monitor the patient closely for signs of drug abuse. Such signs include:

  - selling of prescription drugs or obtaining opioids from unauthorized sources;

  - obtaining opioids from multiple physicians;

  - multiple unsanctioned increases in dose;

  - loss of prescriptions;

  - frequent visits to emergency departments.

- Small numbers of breakthrough doses should be allowed and monitored closely.

Chronic non-malignant pain is far from being benign. Appropriate therapy of such pain can reduce patient suffering and improve quality of life for patients who otherwise may be quite disabled by inadequate pain management.

References

1. Taylor H, Curran NM. *Nuprin Pain Report*. Louis Harris and Associates. New York 1985.

2. Melzack R. The tragedy of needless pain. *Sci Am* 1990; 262:27-33.

3. *Acute Pain Management: Operative and Medical Procedures and Trauma*. U.S. Department of Health and Human Services, Public Health Service, Agency for Health Policy and Research, Washington D.C. February 1992.

4. Portenoy RK. Opioid therapy for chronic nonmalignant pain: a review of the critical issues. *J Pain Sympt Manage* 1996; 11:203-17.

5. Zenz M, Strumpf M, Tryba M. Long-term oral opioid therapy in patients with chronic non-malignant pain. *J Pain Sympt Manage* 1992; 7:69-77.

6. Arkinstall W, Sandler A, Goughnour B et al. Efficacy of controlled-release codeine in chronic non-malignant pain: a randomized, placebo-controlled clinical trial. *Pain* 1995; 62:169-78.

7. Moulin DE, Iezzi A, Amireh R et al. Randomized trial of oral morphine for chronic non-cancer pain. *Lancet* 1996; 347:143-7.

8. Hagen N, Flynne P, Hays H, MacDonald N. Guidelines for managing non-malignant pain. *Can Fam Phys* 1995; 41:49-53.

Appendix A

SYMPTOM ASSESSMENT GRAPH

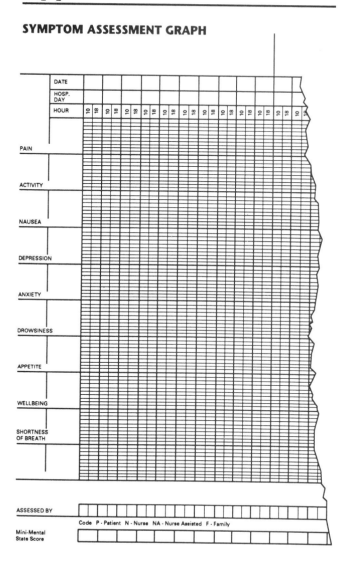

	DATE																							
	HOSP. DAY																							
	HOUR	10	18	10	18	10	18	10	18	10	18	10	18	10	18	10	18	10	18	10	18	10	18	10

PAIN

ACTIVITY

NAUSEA

DEPRESSION

ANXIETY

DROWSINESS

APPETITE

WELLBEING

SHORTNESS OF BREATH

ASSESSED BY

Code   P - Patient   N - Nurse   NA - Nurse Assisted   F - Family

Mini-Mental State Score

SYMPTOM ASSESSMENT GRAPH (cont'd)

Name: _____

Room #: _____ Time: _____

Please cross the line at the point that best describes: (For coding)

No pain _____ Worst possible pain

Not tired _____ Worst possible tiredness

Not nauseated _____ Worst possible nausea

Not depressed _____ Worst possible depression

Not anxious _____ Worst possible anxiety

Not drowsy _____ Worst possible drowsiness

Best possible appetite _____ No appetite

Best possible sensation of wellbeing _____ Worst possible sensation of wellbeing

No shortness of breath _____ Worst possible shortness of breath

_____

Assessed by: _____

Adapted from Bruera E, Kuehn N, Miller MJ et al. The Edmonton Symptom Assessment Scale: A simple method for the assessment of palliative care patients. *J Palliative Care* 1991; 7(2):6-9. With permission.

PAIN REPORT FORM/DIARY

Managing Your Pain

When answering the questions; "How severe was the pain?" and "Did it help?", use the keys to the right as a guide.

A sample entry is provided below.

KEY FOR SEVERITY
(How severe was the pain?)

1	2	3	4	5
Mild	Discomforting	Distressing	Horrible	Excruciating

KEY FOR PAIN RELIEF
(Did it help?)

1	2	3	4	5
No relief	Slight relief	Moderate relief	Lots of relief	Complete relief

When did the pain begin? What was I doing?	How long did it last?	Where was it?	How severe was it? (Rate 1-5) What did it feel like? (e.g., throbbing, steady, sharp, dull, burning, other) What made it worse?	What did I do for relief?	Did it help? (Rate 1-5) Any side effects?
DATE					
9:00 a.m. Eating	1 hour	My chest	2. Throbbing	Took pain medication. Listened to music.	5. No side effects.
DATE					

Adapted from *The 1st Step* booklet, Canadian Cancer Society. With permission

Appendix B

Resources for Pain Control

Palliative Care Resources

a) Patients may consult **The Canadian Palliative Care Association** (**CPCA**) for information about local, regional or provincial palliative care services and programs in their area:

> The Canadian Palliative Care Association
> 286-43 Bruyère Street
> Ottawa, Ontario
> K1N 5C8
> Telephone: 1 800 668-2785
> or (613) 241-3663
> Fax: (613) 562-4226

b) Most provinces have provincial palliative care associations. Telephone numbers are available through the CPCA. Patients may consider joining these associations to take advantage of special continuing education programs sponsored by these organizations.

c) Consult the author of this manual if you wish:

> Dr. Larry Librach
> Division of Palliative Medicine
> Mount Sinai Hospital
> 600 University Avenue
> Toronto, Ontario
> M5G 1X5
> Telephone: (416) 586-8594
> Fax: (416) 586-4804
> e-mail: larry.librach@utoronto.ca

Pain Clinics

a)   Many cancer centres now have cancer pain specialists in medicine and nursing.

b)   Pain clinics for chronic non-malignant pain are often located in university medical centres. A telephone consultation may be all that is required. Waiting lists can be quite long.

Bibliography

Books, Articles and Monographs

American Pain Society. *Principles of Analgesic Use in the Treatment of Acute Pain and Cancer Pain.* (3rd ed.), 1992.

Babul N, Darke AC. Evaluation and use of opioid analgesics in paediatric cancer pain. *J Palliative Care* 1993; 9:9-25.

Doyle D, Hanks GWC, MacDonald N (ed.) *Oxford Textbook of Palliative Medicine.* Oxford Medical Publications, Oxford University Press, Oxford, New York, Tokyo 1993.

Ferris FD, Flannery J. (eds.) *HIV Module 4: Palliative Care, A Comprehensive Guide for the Care of Persons with HIV disease.* Mount Sinai Hospital and Casey House Hospice, Toronto, 1995.

Hanks GW. Morphine sans Morpheus. *Lancet* 1995; 346:652.

Jacox A, Can DB, Payne R et al. *Management of Pain, Clinical Practice Guidelines.* No. 9. A HCPR Publication No. 94-0592. Rockville, MD. Agency for Health Care Policy and Research. US Dept. of Health and Human Services, Public Health Service, 1994.

Kaye P. *Notes on Symptom Control in Hospice & Palliative Care.* Hospice Education Institute (Revised 1st ed.), USA Version, Essex, Connecticut, USA 1990.

Kuttner L. *A Child in Pain: How to Help, What to Do.* Hartley & Marks, Vancouver, 1996.

MacCaffery M and Beebe A. *Pain: A Clinical Manual for Nursing Practice*, CV Mosby, Toronto, 1989.

McGuire D, Yarbo C, Ferrell B. *Cancer Pain Management.* Jones and Bartlett, Boston, 1995.

Murphy GP, Lawrence W, Lenhard RE (ed.) *American Cancer Society Textbook of Clinical Oncology.* (2nd ed.) American Cancer Society, Atlanta, 1995.

Patt RB. *Cancer Pain.* J.B. Lippincott Company, Philadelphia, 1993.

Rando TA. *Grief, Dying and Death: Clinical Interventions for Caregivers.* Research Press Company, Champaign, Illinois, 1984.

Twycross RW and Lack S. *Symptom Control in Far Advanced Cancer: Pain Relief.* Pitman, London, 1984.

Twycross RW and Lack SA. *Therapeutics in Terminal Cancer.* (2nd ed.) Churchill Livingstone, New York, 1990.

Vaino A, Ollila J, Matikanien et al. Driving ability in cancer patients receiving long-term morphine analgesia. *Lancet* 1995; 346:667-70.

Von Roenn J, Cleeland CS, Gonin R. Physician attitudes and practice in cancer pain management. *Ann Inter Med* 1993; 119:121-6.

Wall PD, Melzack R. (ed.) *Textbook of Pain.* Churchill Livingstone, Edinburgh, London, Melbourne and New York, 1992.

World Health Organization. *Cancer Pain and Palliative Care.* World Health Organization Office of Publications, Technical Report, No. 804, Geneva, 1990.

World Health Organization. *Cancer Pain Relief.* World Health Organization Office of Publications, Geneva, 1986.

Recommended Journals

Clinical Journal of Pain

European Journal of Palliative Care

Journal of Pain and Symptom Management

Journal of Palliative Care

Pain

Palliative Medicine

Index